Sleep Monsters and Superheroes

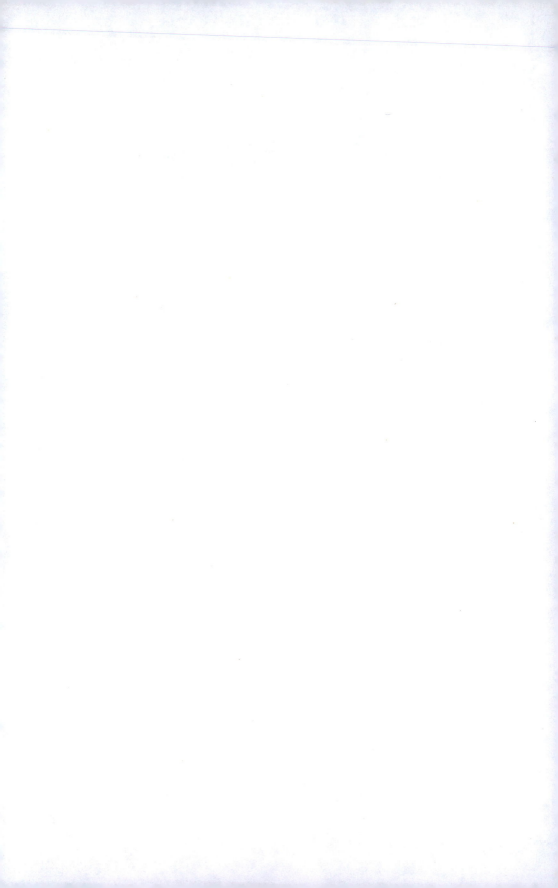

Sleep Monsters and Superheroes

Empowering Children through Creative Dreamplay

Clare R. Johnson and Jean M. Campbell, Editors

Foreword by Deirdre Barrett

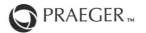 PRAEGER™

An Imprint of ABC-CLIO, LLC
Santa Barbara, California • Denver, Colorado

Library of Congress Cataloging-in-Publication Data

Names: Johnson, Clare R., editor. | Campbell, Jean M., editor.
Title: Sleep monsters and superheroes : empowering children through creative
    dreamplay / Clare R. Johnson and Jean M. Campbell, editors.
Description: Santa Barbara : Praeger, 2016. | Includes bibliographical references
    and index.
Identifiers: LCCN 2016023492 (print) | LCCN 2016033409 (ebook) | ISBN
    9781440842665 (hardcopy : alk. paper) | ISBN 9781440842672 (ebook)
Subjects: LCSH: Children's dreams. | Child psychology. | Creative ability in children.
Classification: LCC BF1099.C55 S555 2016 (print) | LCC BF1099.C55 (ebook)
    | DDC 154.6/3083—dc23
LC record available at https://lccn.loc.gov/2016023492

ISBN: 978–1–4408–4266–5
EISBN: 978–1–4408–4267–2

20 19 18 17 16   1 2 3 4 5

This book is also available as an eBook.

Praeger
An Imprint of ABC-CLIO, LLC

ABC-CLIO, LLC
130 Cremona Drive, P.O. Box 1911
Santa Barbara, California 93116-1911
www.abc-clio.com

This book is printed on acid-free paper ∞

Manufactured in the United States of America

Children are the future.
For intrepid young dreamers all around the world
And for the adults who help them.

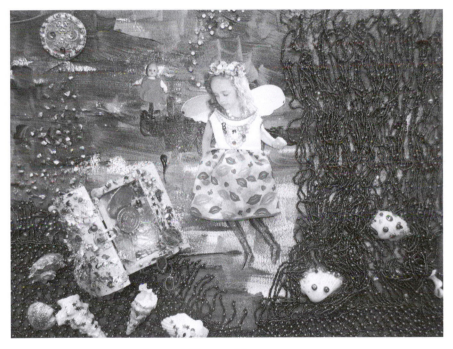

"Finding Treasure in my Dream" (Yasmin Johnson, 6)

Contents

Foreword

Anyone who has children in their lives—parents, teachers, or child therapists, will find *Sleep Monsters and Superheroes: Empowering Children through
Creative Dreamplay* a remarkable resource. This book covers common
dreams, transcendent ones, garden-variety nightmares and the haunted
ones of traumatized children.

There is a scholarly richness: Jung's theories about children's dreams,
how Piagetian developmental stages relate, and the latest findings on the
effects of digital media use on children's dreams are all discussed. However,
the main focus is what most readers will want: practical techniques for helping children get the most out of their dreams. Each chapter introduces
methods by which they can learn about themselves or transform bad
dreams into mastery and creativity.

If you've ever wondered how to comfort a frightened child without
invoking "it's just a dream," there are numerous approaches from verbal
ones to concrete rituals. Similarly, there are many examples of getting children to appreciate metaphors at ages when they couldn't talk about metaphor as a concept. Several chapters describe child dream groups in which
they interact with each other's dreams. Techniques like Gestalt Therapy dialogues take on a new relevance when combined with children's natural pro-
pensity for acting at being various characters. Some chapter authors
specialize in child psychology while others describe the child-appropriate
version of their other specialties such as mastering lucid dreaming or overcoming post-traumatic nightmares.

A unifying concept throughout the book is using play as the royal road to
children's dreams. Storytelling, drawing, making masks of dream characters,
dialoging with characters, and acting out dreams are employed to engage children with dreams. With almost equal emphasis to the techniques adults can

introduce to children, authors repeatedly give examples about simply not getting in the way of children's instinctive sense of the importance of dreams and empathically listening to how kids are already relating to their dreams.

Readers of this book were once children ourselves, so the rich dream accounts scattered throughout will serve to remind us how enchanting childhood dreams can be—fictional friends and superheroes spring to life—and also will invoke how immersively terrifying nightmares are at that age. It will make you wish you'd had these authors around when you were a child waking up eager to recount a wondrous dream or nightmare. But the main function of the book will be to help readers become that person to whom children rush to share their dreams.

Deirdre Barrett, PhD
Cambridge, MA
April 2016

Preface

One day, Clare's four-year-old built a home made from hairbands, feathers, and bits of knitting for her invisible playmate, a pink fairy armadillo.

"That's his safe place," she said.

When Clare had admired it, she asked Yasmin, "Where's *your* safe place?" thinking she would say it was her play-tent, or her bedroom.

But Yasmin replied: "It's you, Mummy—and Daddy, too."

What an awesome gift and responsibility, to be a child's safe place. Family, friends, caregivers, teachers, social workers, and therapists can all offer a sense of safety to children.

So can dreams.

One of the most moving statements in this book—which is packed with deeply human stories—appears in the chapter on traumatized adolescents, where for two teenagers "the experience of safety and love occurred for the first time in their life in their dreams." The magnitude of this statement is enormous. If anybody dismisses dreams as the meaningless, random results of neurons firing in the brain, let's share that story with them, and many others from this book.

Inside *Sleep Monsters and Superheroes*, there are stories about dreams that help children fight cancer; dreams that empower children to face moments of great change; spiritual dreams of transcendence. If just one dream can give a child solace after bereavement or self-worth after abuse, then what might be possible when we help children to work and play with their dreams on a regular basis?

Dreamplay can be defined as working and playing with a dream for therapy, empowerment, creativity, or fun—and sometimes all of these at the same time. Each chapter has a practical section to make it useful for parents, caregivers, health professionals, educators, and therapists.

These practical techniques help adults to help children with dreams, nightmares, and waking life issues. When children improve their dream life and access valuable unconscious resources, their waking life tends to become correspondingly happier because they feel empowered to act—and react—in new ways.

Our highly experienced, hardworking team of authors have created inspiring chapters and shared their most useful dreamplay tips to help adults to accompany children as they unwrap their dream gifts of healing, wisdom, and inner resources. The first part, "Creativity and Healing," is made up of four chapters: first, Patricia Garfield gives insights into the symbolic language of dreams and shows how young children can turn their dreams into creative adventures. Nightmares and their creative and healing potential are then discussed by Kelly Bulkeley and Patricia M. Bulkley, followed by our jointly written chapter on the power of storytelling to transform the dream life of children of all ages. The final chapter in this section is by Tallulah Lyons, who considers the ways in which dreamplay can help children facing illness, injury, and physical handicaps.

Part Two, "Inner and Outer Worlds," begins with Angel Morgan's chapter, which examines children's inner worlds through the universal language of their dreams. Jayne Gackenbach and her students then take a close look at the way current digital technology impacts children's dreams, and Martha Taylor explores children's outer worlds through the influence of community on their dreams.

"Extreme Dreams" are the subject of Part Three: David Gordon and Dani Vedros show how dreams can help adolescents who have suffered from trauma and difficult life circumstances. Their chapter is followed by Brenda Mallon's insights into the dreams of bereaved and grieving children. Ryan Hurd then discusses "weird" nighttime experiences such as night terrors and disorders in children's sleep, and the section closes with Jean Campbell's examination of the ways in which war affects children's dreams, and how we can dream a peaceful world into being.

In Part Four, the book moves from extreme dreams into "Extraordinary Dreams." Linda Mastrangelo investigates the dreams of time, space, and the future that young dreamers can experience, and Kate Adams dives into the divine in her chapter on religious and spiritual themes in children's dreams. The final chapter, by Clare Johnson, explores the ways in which children can be empowered through lucid dreaming.

Sleep Monsters and Superheroes takes the reader on a journey into the empowerment of children through dreamplay. This book shows how all these different types of dreams and life situations can be turned around through dreamplay to help a child to gain inner resources such as resilience, healing from trauma, and the fearless acceptance of scary but necessary things like hospital visits. In the pages of this book, we discover who the monsters are that terrorize our children at night, and how we can help children to cope with nightmares by transforming them into creative, healing play. Led into dreamplay by a supportive adult, children can become "superheroes" in their dreams, and this empowerment carries over into their waking lives.

> Children are our future.
> Dreamplay can empower children to have stronger inner resources and happier lives.
> Let's help children to open the door to their dreams.

We wish you and the children you care for creative and empowering dreams!

Clare R. Johnson and Jean M. Campbell

PART ONE
Creativity and Healing

CHAPTER ONE

Superkid and Other Joyful Dreams: Creative Dreaming with Young Children[1]

Patricia Garfield

I am Superboy flying through the air. And I'm looking for a bad guy's sailboat.
Adam, age eight

"Sweet dreams!" many parents say to their children at bedtime. Now and then, sandwiched between scary and frustrating nightmares, children do indeed have very pleasant dreams. In a study I did of the dreams reported by 120 children aged five to twelve (58 boys and 62 girls), I found that most of the 288 dreams collected were frightening (158); less were positive (89); even less were unclassifiable (41).[2]

Good dreams satisfy a multitude of children's needs. Since antiquity, thoughtful people such as Sigmund Freud have observed that some types of dreams fulfill a wish.[3] When my daughter, at about seven years, dreamed of coming downstairs to find a set of yellow sneakers waiting for her, she presented herself with the object of her desire. Other pleasurable dreams express needs or wishes that are more abstract. While they are quite young, middle-class children in many cultures develop a need to achieve. They are urged to get good grades, to excel in sports, to develop musical, artistic, or dancing skills. Psychologists find that children coming from homes where they are encouraged to solve problems at an early age and to become independent are those who acquire a strong need for achievement.[4] This need is clearly expressed in some of children's happy dreams.

All of us want our efforts to yield accomplishment. Yet children who set goals much higher than the level they are capable of are doomed to disappointment; they may be trying to attain goals their parents and peers have set, instead of their own. Conversely, children who set goals well below their ability to achieve have perhaps learned to fear failure and so try to avoid it. Researchers tell us that people who have a sense of accomplishment in life are those who set goals just *a little beyond the level they are sure to attain.* As parents, we can assist our children in setting realistic goals; we can glimpse these inner goals through the window of our children's dreams.

By tuning in to your child's dream life, you become capable of seeing what needs are developing and what shapes the sources of their pleasure take. If your child has few or no pleasant dreams, this chapter provides suggestions for promoting them. Happy dreams do more than make a wish come true. They give solace for a miserable day; they refresh and revive sagging spirits; they offer a chance to practice skills in art and sport as well as ideas for new creations. Pleasant dreams make children feel important and loved. They stir a sense of adventure, bring a touch of magic; even give a glimmer of the mystical. Moreover, having good dreams is fun—your child needs them.

My mother's interest in dreams inspired my own; I started a dream diary at the age of fourteen that continues to this day. I came to understand more about myself through this long-term dream record. When I traveled widely around the world I learned how much different cultures influence dream content. These experiences inspired me to put together a book on the subject of dreams that could be used for my psychology students in the university where I taught. The book *Creative Dreaming*, first published in 1974, became a classic. I dedicated my professional life to the study of how dreams can help dreamers to lead more fulfilling lives and went on to write a total (so far) of 12 books on dreams, including *Your Child's Dreams* in 1984, and most recently in 2015, *Schmoopie's Dream.* Now, with my 81st birthday behind me, I remain convinced of the enduring power and importance of dreams in a person's life.

As I sorted the happy dreams in my study, I found, as with nightmares, the dreams involved a limited number of themes. In this chapter, I will look at dreams of media heroes, desirable possessions, magical animal friends, loving and flying dreams, and more, to give a full picture of children's joyful dreams. I will then provide practical suggestions for working—and playing—with children's dreams.

Superkid: The Media Hero

The superhero or superheroine represents a deep desire children have for more control over their lives. Perhaps because boys and girls are so much smaller and less powerful than the adults around them, tales of the super-hero have always been popular. From Samson in the Bible to Hercules in myths of old, from the Lone Ranger and Superman to Yoda in films, car-toons, and comics, children yearn for a powerful figure on whom they can pin their hopes for overcoming difficulties. Such figures help children evolve their own mastery.

Characters who can accomplish the impossible are very useful for chil-dren at a certain stage of development. They provide fantasy figures on whom they can focus their daydreams as well as their night dreams. If child-ren's obsession with superheroes endures into adolescence, however, and if fictional heroes and heroines are not gradually replaced by living men and women who have managed to make contributions of value, the youngster is left adrift in a sea of fantasy.

The superhero figures in our mass media tend to overemphasize physical power, even violence, in accomplishing their feats of heroism. As parents, we can augment our children's supply of heroes and heroines by sharing stories, legends, and films that portray a variety of outstanding people, fic-tional and real, with a range of skills beyond solely superhuman strength.

If your child dreams of a superhero, he or she is reaching for the strength of this character, for the pleasure of being able to do well and of being rec-ognized for it. A few children in my study, like Adam in his dream of "Superboy" at the start of this chapter, reveled in the powers of the media superhero. They possessed inordinate strength; they flew. Eight-year-old Kevin also cast himself as Superman, adding male savior:

> *I had a dream that I was Superman saving Lois Lane. And she was hanging on the Golden Gate Bridge. Then she fell but I came. Then I grabbed her and brought her home.*

Aaron, almost five, played out the same pleasant fantasy in a slightly different version:

> *Superman was my dad. He really was my dad. He was not the dad that is my dad in this real life. My mom was Supergirl.*

When asked, "What happened? What did they do?" Aaron replied, "Super-parents!" Since his own parents are divorced, one cannot help but wonder whether Aaron is wishing for some improved model parents in his dream.

In a scary dream he had around the same time, Aaron dreamed that Superman rescued him from a closet. He clearly felt a need for help.

Jason, age six, added a second superhero to his nighttime adventure:

> *Yesterday I dreamed that I was in TV. I was in Superfiend. I was Batman. Then I saw Superman in a cake with a coconut. Then I went to break the coconut so Superman could run out and fly. Then I got up.*

In Jason's version it was the dreamer who had the capacity to release Superman, who was trapped inside a coconut like a genie in a bottle. Charmaine, age eight, put herself in the part of a traditional superheroine:

> *Last night I dreamed that I was Wonder Woman. And I threw bad people in prison.*

The Superkid theme was relatively rare in my study (7 of 288 dreams). If your child should have frequent dreams about being a superhero, chances are that the child is reaching for strength, achievement, importance, and self-reliance.

Heroes and Heroines: Outstanding Performances

Slightly more popular than Superkid dreams were dreams of more or less mortal heroes and heroines who performed some fantastic dream accomplishment (9 of 288 dreams). For example, Eric, age eight, said:

> *The dream had excitement, adventure, danger, and thrills. I was a hero. I saved the princess from the Duke. She was guarded by a dragon. The dragon was killed and then the Duke came out! I fought him. I won the battle. I took her back to the king and then we got married and then we became king and queen and we lived happily ever after.*

As in a classical fairy tale, Eric as hero defended the princess, won, and married her. Although defeating a dragon is a superhuman task, the hero was pictured as a normal person, suggesting this child's need for achievement may be realistic.

Genevieve, age eleven, reported a pleasant dream of possessing power by supernatural means:

> *I'm supposed to be a good witch that makes people happy. What I see in the picture [she was describing the drawing she had done of her dream] is that I'm making a girl real small and she's floating. I don't know the girl. There is a live tree, a live sun and also a live cat around me. A real little girl that's floating and there's a*

big, big mouse. And a bird that's climbing up a tree. This is happening around a neighbor's house.

Elizabeth, age six, drew on a mythical female for her achievement:

Last night I dreamed about I was a mermaid in the ocean. Then I went to a pool. I swam around the pool, staying underwater for five minutes. Then I came up and rested for a while.

Your child's interests are almost sure to show up in dreams, especially of achieving a victory in a game. Boys and girls who enjoy athletics perform great feats in their happy dreams, conferring the status of hero.

Seth, age six, excelled in the field of dream running:

I liked my race and it was fun and I won it. I saw an ambulance pass by.

Some awareness of danger was present, in the ambulance, but Seth achieved his goal nonetheless.

Jenna, age eleven, like Seth, won a jogging race in her dreams:

I was running in the Bay to Breakers [a local race]. At the last hill, two winners came in. I was first in children, and the first female, but third including the men.

Although Jenna placed herself in the forefront of women and children in skill, she rated herself lower than the best men, a view that could limit her ability to achieve. Another girl, eight-year-old Mikele, made her great performance in the schoolyard:

I dreamt that I was a great monkey bars swinger. (But I'm not.)

Children sometimes accomplish something remarkable in their dreams by winning a contest or by being chosen for a special role. Eight-year-old Tara, for instance, dreamed:

At the end of class, I was chosen to sing a solo. A smile grew on my face. Our teacher said, "Thank you for a wonderful rehearsal." I ran out to tell my mom I had been chosen for a solo. She was very pleased—so was I.

Tara actually takes singing lessons, so this dream is likely to be a kind of practice, a behavioral rehearsal for waking-life events, as well as a wishful expression of a desire for recognition. Jenna, too, age eleven, actually performs in her daily life. Her singing and acting often appear in her dreams, reflecting this lively interest. In one:

I was a singer and I got nominated for the Grammys [a recording award]. So I sang my song and it wasn't me. I was disappointed. Then I found out it was the wrong category. But I won the real category.

A relative of Jenna's recently won a Grammy award, so this wishful dream is realistically possible in the child's mind. In another dream, Jenna played the heroine in the movie *Grease*. Jenna's frequent dreams about performing reveal vivid interest in her activities and her dream practice helps her prepare to do well.

Helen Keller, when an undergraduate at Radcliffe College, dreamed that she was Napoleon astride a fiery steed on top of a hill, surveying her army. As her men surged across the green fields to the sound of trumpets, drums, and marching feet, Helen/Napoleon charged with sword held high. Throwing herself furiously into dream battle, she struck the bedpost and awoke.[5] The role of the conqueror in Helen's dream probably depicted her enormous struggle to surmount her handicaps of blindness and deafness in obtaining a college degree. Few dreamers would feel themselves to be Napoleon; yet in terms of Helen's personal accomplishment, the role was apt.

Children's dreams of outstanding performance provide opportunities to taste victory, to stretch talents, and to practice skills. The child succeeds and is rewarded for it. These dreams help shape self-confidence. If your child reports dreams of being a superhero or of making an outstanding performance, you can be fairly certain the child has developed a need for achievement. Help your child to establish worthwhile goals in the same range as his or her abilities.

Being Important

Related to dreams of superheroes and outstanding performances are dreams of being important. In these, however, the dreamer does nothing to merit distinction; the role is simply provided: the dreamer *is* important. For example, Kenric, age eight, stated:

Yesterday I dreamt of Star Trek. *Then I thought I was Captain of the* Enterprise.

In a similar spirit, eight-year-old Mira dreamed of being an actress; Kimberly cast herself as actor. When children visualize themselves as important without describing the behavior involved in achieving this status, they may not yet realize how to achieve goals in life. If your child reports such dreams, show that you understand the desire by comments like

"How did that feel? That must have been fun. It sounds like a great adventure." You may wish to follow up with a discussion of how to achieve occupations of the sort mentioned. "Maybe someday you would like to study acting. To be a captain, you need to do a good job in the armed service," and so on. Help the child understand the connection between prominence and personal effort.

Aside from having a military rank or being on stage, children bestow importance on themselves in dreams by becoming royalty. A few girls in my study mentioned dreams of being a princess, drawing pictures of themselves in crown and royal robes. Five-year-old Aaron dreamed his mother was a princess and he a prince in classic Freudian style (where a male child desires to marry his mother). Six-year-old Banner became regent by gift of a magical creature:

> *This elf saw me and he got me a king's hat [a crown] and he made me king of the palace. And everybody that was bad is put in there.*

If your child has this dream theme, you might say, "Sometimes it's fun to pretend we are very important and can do what we want to do. There are other ways to get what we want, too." At the same time, allow your child to enjoy fulfilling fantasies. Encourage your child to understand that being famous usually requires preparations and solid work. Those children who "earn" their importance—by practice or effort—are likely to be outstanding achievers in waking life, as well. They work to produce their accomplishments in dreams just as they do while awake.

I wish, I wish, I wish . . . Dreams about Desirable Possessions

Children often dream of the wonderful things they want to have. In these dreams, parents can see the values their children are developing and the subjects that preoccupy their minds. Such dreams give the dreamer pleasure whether or not they ever acquire in waking life the object dreamed about. Adults dream of desirable possessions less often, perhaps because money is more readily available to purchase some of the objects of their dreams. As children mature, the "goods" that seem most appealing to them shift.

These marvelous objects are sometimes gifts, as second grader Michael reported:

> *My dream was about Santa giving me a CB [citizen's band radio transmitter] and I play with it.*

Eight-year-old Maya received her dream gift from a magical bug:

> *One day when I was coming home, suddenly [I met] a little Ladybug and it gave*
> *me a wish. I asked my mom what I should wish for. She said,*
> *"A color TV with everlasting tube."*
> *"Okay."*
> *"Oh bug, oh bug."*
> *"Yes?"*
> *"My wish is I want a color TV."*
> *"There you go."*
> *"Wow!"*

Wealth is the sought-after possession in certain dreams. Eight-year-old Kimberly, for example, reported:

> *Last night I dreamed that I was a millionaire and I had maids and servants and I*
> *lived in a mansion and I was happy.*

The underlying wish in such dreams seems to be for a freedom to do whatever the dreamer wants, including buying anything in the world. Sometimes the dreamer's object of desire is an instrument. Five-year-old Eric dreamed:

> *Mother and I were in the woods. I call Mother's attention to a bow and arrow.*
> *I show it to her and ask her how to use it. She shows me.*

From a psychoanalytic viewpoint, the bow and arrow of Eric's dream, in addition to being an object he wishes to have, may also symbolize the penis that the child is learning how to use properly. Psychoanalytically, dream instruments represent male sexuality.[6] More generally, such dreams express pleasure in mastering new skills.

On the Good Ship Lollipop: Dreams of Delicious Food

Special food treats are another kind of desirable possession that takes shape in children's dreams. Seven-year-old Kierstin told about going on a picnic with "good food like fruit, meat, and cake." Asgar, a ten-year-old boy from India, reported:

> *I dreamed that eggplants and mangoes came down from heaven with the rain. A*
> *funny, silly dream.*

The type of food that is regarded as scrumptious will vary from country to country. Few American children would look forward to feasting on eggplants and mangoes. Chocolate, ice cream, cupcakes, and cake seem to be universally desirable. Anne, age seven, dreamed of 5,000 gallons of cherry ice cream with a cherry on top; Robyn, at eight, remembered a dream from age four of a strawberry ice-cream cone that "went on and on and on." A little girl from India, seven-year-old Shalina, described her "sweet dream":

> *I saw that I am wandering in my beautiful garden and suddenly I see many chocolates hanging out of the trees. I start eating them.*

Eight-year-old Amit, a boy from India, dreamed:

> *The ice cream seller is shouting, "Come, children, come, have wonderful ice cream," in the lane outside my house.*

Dreams of food can reflect hunger, as researchers find in the dreams of deprived and starving people. In psychoanalytic theory, dreaming of food is thought to reflect dependency needs—the oral gratification associated with need for love. Food comes to represent satisfaction of emotional needs for affection.[7] If your child reports many dreams of food, you might ask yourself whether the child is receiving enough physical and emotional nourishment.

Happy Days in Dreamland: Pleasurable Dream Activities

For adults, holidays are usually symbolic: Dreams of Christmas to mark a special emotional event; dreams of Easter to accompany a sense of an emotional rebirth; dreams of *Yom Kippur* (the Jewish Day of Atonement) may represent a sense of guilt, and so on. Children are more likely to be dreaming of the delight a holiday brings—freedom from schoolwork, the chance for games, trips, gifts, and good food. Jeremy, for instance, said: *I dreamed it was Halloween. I was a wizard and went trick-or-treating.* Since Jeremy had this dream in March, it was not likely to be anticipatory of the October holiday. Perhaps he felt special in some wizard-like or tricky way. In some of their dreams, children rejoice in a plain, ordinary, lovely day. Seven-year-old Petrina, for example, stated: *I had a dream about a beautiful day with flowers and butterflies flying in the sky.* Flying creatures, animal or human, are often associated with dreams that feel magical to children. Petrina's dream is characteristic of a happy mood, when things seem to be going especially well or the dreamer feels encouraged.

An older girl, eleven-year-old Devon, dreamed:

> *When I was walking in the park, there was a rainbow and then there was a light in back of it, a whole bunch. They called it a rainbow rally. I kept asking people why*

there were so many rainbows. They didn't answer me. I guess they were just hav-
ing a rainbow day.

    I kept walking and seeing more rainbows; the sky was made of rainbows; the
shops were made of rainbows. Everything was made of rainbows except the house.
The house was made of white and inside everything was made of rainbows.

For children as well as adults, the rainbow is a symbol of joy. Several children in my study included them in happy dreams. Whether one thinks of
the biblical account of God's promise never again to inflict a destructive
flood destroying humankind, or recalls the Irish fairy tales of the pot of gold
at the end of the rainbow or the Indian myth of the rainbow bridge,
the symbol is full of hope. So, too, Devon must have felt hopeful when
she had her dream of a rainbow rally.

    In addition to birthday celebrations and holidays, marriages take place in
sunny dreams. Ten-year-old Asgar from India, said:

I dreamt that my teacher was married in a house. The house had flowers all over
and the candles were lighted. My teacher had a garland on his neck. He was very
cheerful. After [the] marriage, he gave a tea party for me and my friends. It was
very enjoyable. A wonderful dream.

For older children and adults, marriage in a dream may have acquired the
symbolic meaning of union or spiritual alliance.

    Trips, too, are often pleasurable events in dreamland. Children visit rela-
tives, tour beautiful cities, and explore the world in their happy dreams.
A dream Kevin had about being in space and one of Tyler's about a flying
ship are journeys in a higher atmosphere. Phillip, age seven, had a dream
trip reminiscent of Dorothy's in the land of Oz:

Once there was a hurricane and it lifted my house to a strange land. But I woke
up—too bad.

Such dreams reflect the growing child's curiosity about the environment, to
reach out, to experience, and to explore.

    Another form of pleasure in children's dreams is playing games. When
Eric was four, he dreamed:

I have a friend and I play with him in a bathtub. The dream has three parts. First
we played in my playroom. Then we all went upstairs and Mother turned on the
water and we took a bath. Kind of fun.

In India, Amit described several games in his dreams. In one: *I saw that*
I am playing nearby a river and building sand castles! This game I like most.

Stacy, age six, said: *Last night I dreamed about my Barbie dream house and my Barbie doll, too.* Stacy was deliberately attending to her dreams at this time and so may have been influenced to dream of a *dream house*. Although not obviously happy in this dream or obviously playing, it is likely that the little girl is both. She already possessed these desirable objects, so the emphasis is on using them. Celebrations, holidays, trips, games—these pleasurable activities proved to be the most popular category of children's good dreams.

Loving Dreams

Children only rarely expressed loving feelings as the themes of their dreams. Betty, age six, relayed a typical example: *One night I had a dream called, 'Myself.' I love myself and I love my mom and my daddy.* Aaron, age five, told his dream one morning: *I was kissing you [his mother] and there was a bluebird singing in the tree.* A poignant example of a loving dream came from Amit, in India:

> My grandmother [who died recently] is sitting by my bed and singing a song, my favorite, and I am happy, thinking, 'Grandma is back from heaven.'

People often dream of those they loved returning from the dead. These dreams can be extremely painful; sometimes, as with Amit's, they bring exquisite pleasure.

Althea, at about age four, dreamed that hearts were flowing from her mother's mouth. Hearts, a traditional symbol for love, frequently convey this feeling in dreams. When I was in my early teens, I often dreamed of hats shaped like hearts, indicating that my mind was full of thoughts about love. Perhaps because dreams are primarily directed toward dreamers' attempts to solve their problems, the emotion of love is seldom expressed in them. How happy parents must feel to find that their loving concern is recognized at a profound level in their children's dreams.

Flying Dreams

Of all the pleasures a child enjoys in dreams, perhaps the most delightful is being able to fly. Magic carpets, flying ships, and superheroes whizzing through the air have similar appeal. Five-year-old Aaron dreamed:

> I was riding in a car with Judith [a family friend]. I looked out the window and saw some Smurfs [a modern version of the magical elves]. I jumped out of the window and flew up into the sky, as high as the rockets go.

Aaron reported this dream with eyes aglow: "Mom, I made myself do it," (i.e., fly). He was very pleased with the accomplishment. Across the world in India, nine-year-old Amit shared his version of this same blissful dream:

> *I am flying like a bird while the moon is shining and some birds are also awakened and flying with me.*

When she was ten, Jenna added a unique touch to her night flying:

> *I dreamt I am a bird, a beautiful white egret flying in the clouds, and all these bluebirds are around. My feathers blow in the wind as I fly. I wonder how to catch a castle, because it flies around. Some people put me on top of the castle. They give me a spell. The people who give me the spell are angels.*

Jenna, like many children and adults, associates bluebirds with happiness, as in the Maeterlinck play *The Bluebird of Happiness* and the film that was based on it. Although these are before Jenna's time, the expression has become an idiom. Jenna defined birds as creatures who "can be mean or nice; they can hurt; they have feelings; they're very scared." Yet, in her dream, Jenna seems to identify with another part of birds, the one that is free to fly to the realm of the angels. Here the child herself is an animal.

Flying dreams sometimes begin in a nightmare when a child is being attacked and discovers, with astonishment, that it is possible to escape by flying away. This discovery sometimes prevents further bad dreams. One young woman who was lucky enough to realize, as a child, that she could fly in her dreams was puzzled why other children had nightmares. Those who fly in their dreams often derive from them a sense of extraordinary freedom. Children as young as four have described flying dreams to me, despite the claims by some theorists that boys and girls do not fly in their dreams until age nine.[8] For many people, dreams of flying are among the most pleasurable, imparting joy to the dreamer. It is a rare person who tells me dreams of fearfully flying too high or of "landing" with difficulty. In general, flying dreams are pure fun. Flying in dreams is a treasured experience in children's dreams. They find flying a sensuous, delightful dream pastime that borders on the enchanted.

Magical Animal Friends

The pleasant dream that surprised me the most, out of all the ones I anticipated children having, was about animal friends. Accustomed to the terror that most animal dreams provoke, it was a joy to discover that children also frisk playfully through their dreamscapes with magical animal allies. Meeting a miraculous animal friend in dreams proved to be very special to the dreamer.[9] Sometimes when children dream happily about animals, they are simply having fun in their sleep. Six-year-old Tyger's report exemplifies this level:

> *In my dream I had a rabbit to play with and I played with him all the time, every day.*

At other times, children take cheer in watching the free activities of wild creatures in their dreams. Anna, not yet three, told of watching dolphins play in the waves.

Eight-year-old Becky gave her account of a beautiful place complete with a magical beast:

> *I'm dreaming of a unicorn and this is a field and it is running across. There's a thorn bush here [she says of her drawing]. And it keeps running and with its sharp horn it cuts away the thorns and it runs through. The unicorn sniffs flowers. It keeps running and jumping and listening to birds and smelling the fresh air.*

Becky's dream animal is having a grand time; it is able to "cut away" the "thorns" (which probably symbolize difficulties). When I asked her why she thought she had such a happy dream, Becky explained that it was the night of her eighth birthday party and everything had gone well. Becky's unicorn frolics to give shape to her pleasure.

Boys and girls may step beyond watching animals or playing with domestic ones in their dreams. From time to time, they tame the wild creatures. Jimmy, in second grade, said:

> *My dream was about an elephant was coming after me and I gave him a peanut and brung him home.*

By taming a wild animal in a dream, children gain a sense of control over their instincts. They are relating to their "animal side' in a cooperative way. Instead of being terrorized by the beast within, children who relate happily to animals in dreams are transforming their instinctual energy. Rather than dreams of being chased and attacked by wild creatures, indicating what they perceive to be destructive energy (in themselves or people around them), their vital forces are becoming constructive.

When animals talk in children's dreams, when they give aid or counsel or inspire awe, they reveal other levels of the dreaming mind. When Althea was six-and-a-half, she related:

I was going out to play. Then a bunny said, "Hi!" I followed him and I saw a carrot house.

Dream animals may grant wishes: a ladybug gave Maya a color television; a lion gifted Michelle with a bike. Five-year-old Aaron's animal friend showed him around the woods in a dream that suggests sensual awakening:

I was in a forest and I saw a family of unicorns. There was a mother unicorn, a father unicorn, a brother unicorn and a sister unicorn. The mother and father unicorn were married. They were kissing and no one argued. The brother unicorn let me touch his skin and his horn and his feet. And then he took me for a ride. The unicorns were all golden and silver.

Whatever sexual symbolism may be construed in the one-horned animal, Aaron derived a pleasure beyond the ordinary from his wondrous ride with the unicorn and his close contact with this mythological creature of the forest. Aaron was safely led through the unknown (the woods) by his animal guide; this suggests he had a good relationship with his own animal instincts.

Twelve-year-old Amber's dream friend took her into the depths of the ocean:

I went down in the sea on a turtle . . . and went to a palace where I met the queen. I also met a turtle, and he told me his name, but I forgot it. He let me inside his shell! It was beautiful.

Amber's greatest pleasure emanated from a sense of being included in secret, "deep" knowledge. The ocean, like the forest, often symbolizes the unconscious, the realm of the unknown. To relate to the depths positively, to explore it with a friendly guide, is a kind of blessing. No wonder this is Amber's favorite dream.

Animals that talk or teach the dreamer are "archetypes." Ancient peoples regarded these animals that were wise beyond human powers, in dream or vision, as "spirit guides."[10] American Indians sought them in vision quests; shamans derived their power from them. Even today in primitive cultures dream animals are considered holy—especially those who aid or advise the dreamer. You might think of such creatures in your child's dreams as cooperative figures of the dreaming mind, molded from the unconscious.

As parents, we want to do whatever we can to promote positive animal or animal-like figures in our child's dreams. When children are able to establish a friendly relationship with deep levels of their minds, as indicated by helpful dream animals, their own creative resources become more available.

Energy to unfold talents, and inspiration to do so, becomes a nightly possibility.

Parents as Guides to Dreamland: Practical Tips

1. **Scan your child's dream record for positive dreams.** Don't be surprised at finding only a few; children often have more upsetting dreams than happy ones. Here are the categories of positive dream themes, listed in the order of frequency found in children in my study:[11]
   - Enjoying a nice activity (trip, birthday, holiday, pretty day).
   - Obtaining a desirable possession.
   - Giving an outstanding performance.
   - Being important or knowing someone important (royalty, sports star, film star).
   - Having an adventure.
   - Being a superhero or superheroine.
   - Seeing or eating delicious food.
   - Meeting an animal or supernatural friend.
   - Being loved.
   - Flying.

2. **Notice any patterns in your child's pleasant dreams.** For instance, a large number of dreams about food may indicate a preoccupation based on a need either for actual food or for more emotional nurturance. The themes in your child's dreams reveal their interests and/or their needs.

3. **If your child has reported no positive dreams, promote them by trying the following:**
   - **Make a suggestion.** When you tuck your child in bed, try asking, "What will you dream about tonight? What would be fun?" Ask about dreams in the morning so the child realizes you are interested—but do not press.
   - **Provide a model.** Share with your child some funny or joyful dream of your own or tell them about one of the happy dreams reported by children in this chapter. Ask, "Have you ever had a dream like that? It might be fun. You could imagine it happening to you as you fall asleep. You might dream about it."[12]
   - **Read happy stories.** Reading books aloud where the hero or heroine has a good dream adventure can also encourage the child to realize that happy dreams are possible and help generate them. Select stories that involve topics the child would enjoy dreaming about; read them aloud just before the child falls asleep.

4. **Reinforce your child's positive dreams.** Convey to your children the message that their good dreams are important:
   - **Listen to and discuss your child's dreams.**
   - **Draw your child's dreams** (if the child is very young) or ask the child to draw it. Put such drawings in a prominent place.

- **Write stories or poems based on the child's dreams.**
- **Incorporate dream content into daily life.** Any art form or craft is useful. Parents might knit a sweater with a favorite dream motif, decorate a quilt or knit a blanket with many personal dream images—a treasure for the child going to sleep. Parents who do not have the time or inclination to use their child's pleasant dream motifs in art form may accomplish the same purpose by obtaining objects that relate to the dream. For instance, a pin or medallion of the animal friend your child met in a dream will keep him or her in touch with the sense of magic and strength the original dream provided. When worn by the child, a unicorn, an elephant, a turtle, or other dream friend reminds the dreamer of a special experience.

5. **Value your child's good dreams.** Show your child that dreams can be marvelous adventures and great fun, as well as resources for creative work. Child experts tell us that children who are imaginative often have higher intelligence and are better able to cope with life.[13] By promoting your child's pleasant dreams, you are stimulating positive fantasy; you are improving the child's ability to profit from internal experience; and you are helping the child to learn to cope with life. By teaching the concepts of transforming dreams to face dangers in bad dreams; getting help when necessary; and using imagination to promote positive dreaming, you may well accelerate your child's process of psychological growth.

Dreaming for a Happier Life

Although children's negative dreams dominate, happy dreams do appear. Along with everyday wish fulfillment, children with these joyful dreams seem to express a yearning that is near mystical. They talk with the animals, become one with them, fly to the stars, and share in the secrets of the universe. These pleasurable dreams bring happiness to our children. Instead of tears, they awaken with shining eyes to tell of adventures.

How can we help our offspring and students move from dreams of despair to dreams of joy? How can the perilous sea of nightmares be crossed? It is possible to move from the common bad dreams to the shores of happier dreamlands. By developing different patterns of dreaming we can help our children become happier. In turn, their dreams have a positive influence on their lives. Children can exercise and expand their creative talents and use their dreams in beneficial ways. The journey is not easy, but it is full of self-discovery and growth.

Notes

1. Originally published in *Your Child's Dreams*, © Garfield 1978. Revised 2015.
2. Patricia Garfield, *Your Child's Dreams* (New York: Ballantine, 1984). See Appendix A: 385–394 for results of Garfield's study. Note: The majority (109) of the children were American; the minority (11) were from Varanasi, India.
3. Sigmund Freud, *The Interpretation of Dreams*, trans. A. A. Brill (New York: Modern Library, 1994), 42–43.
4. Dorothy Corkille Briggs, *Your Child's Self-Esteem* (Garden City, New York: Doubleday & Co., 1975), 257–259.
5. Helen Keller, *The Story of My Life* (New York: Dell, 1980), 404–406.
6. Emil Gutheil, *The Handbook of Dream Analysis* (New York: Liveright Publishing Corporation, 1970), 136–139.
7. Norman Cameron, *Personality Development and Psychopathology* (Boston: Houghton Mifflin, 1963), 39–60 and 427–430.
8. C. W. Kimmins, *Children's Dreams* (London: George Allen & Unwin, Ltd. 1937), quoted in Gutheil, *Handbook of Dream Analysis*, 481.
9. Cameron, *Personality Development.*
10. Claude Lévi-Strauss, *Totemism* (Boston: Beacon Press, 1963), 18–23.
11. Garfield, *Your Child's Dreams.*
12. Ibid.
13. Briggs, *Your Child's Self-Esteem.*

Bibliography

Cameron, Norman. *Personality Development and Psychopathology.* Boston: Houghton Mifflin, 1963.

Corkille Briggs, Dorothy. *Your Child's Self-Esteem.* Garden City, New York: Doubleday & Co., 1975.

Freud, Sigmund. *The Interpretation of Dreams.* Translated by Dr. A. A. Brill. New York: Modern Library, 1994.

Garfield, Patricia. *Your Child's Dreams.* New York: Ballantine, 1984.

Gutheil, Emil. *The Handbook of Dream Analysis.* New York: Liveright Publishing Corporation, 1970.

Keller, Helen. *The Story of My Life.* New York: Dell, 1980.

Kimmins, C. W. *Children's Dreams.* London: George Allen & Unwin, Ltd., 1937.

Lévi-Strauss, Claude. *Totemism.* Boston: Beacon Press, 1963.

CHAPTER TWO

Nightmares as a Gift: The Surprising Value of Frightening Dreams in Childhood

Kelly Bulkeley and Patricia M. Bulkley

Your body starts moving out of bed before you are fully awake and aware of what is happening. Your child is crying nearby, calling for you, obviously very, very scared. You stagger forward in the darkness, blinking your eyes as your own primal fear reaction sets in. Your mind is filled with a single urgent idea—your child is in some kind of danger, and you have to do something about it.

For most parents their introduction to the subject of children's dreams comes in the middle of the night, when they are suddenly awakened by cries of distress from their child. Almost all children have bad dreams and nightmares at some point during their early lives, so this becomes a standard question of healthy child-rearing: What should a parent do in that middle-of-the-night situation? What is the best way to respond to children who have nightmares? What can be done to help children make sense of these upsetting dreams and constructively process the fears they generate?

A nightmare can be defined as an extremely frightening or upsetting dream that wakes the person up, often with carryover feelings of distress. People in cultures all over the world have reported dreams with these qualities,[1] and modern researchers have helped illuminate some of the basic psychological patterns found in frightening dreams.[2] Their work supports a practical approach that recognizes nightmares as a normal and natural part of human life, particularly early in child development.

As a son-and-mother author team, our interest in this topic has a kind of mirror relationship to the subject of our previous work together, *Dreaming Beyond Death: A Guide to Pre-Death Dreams and Visions*. That book focused on dreaming experience at the very end of the life cycle, as people anticipate death and whatever lies beyond. After finishing that work we wondered what it would be like to do a project together on dreams at the very beginning of the life cycle, meaning the earliest remembered dreams of childhood. This was an appealing path to follow because it allowed us to combine our interest in Jungian psychology with our personal experiences as parents and members of an extended family of dream-sharers. The result was our 2012 book *Children's Dreams: Understanding the Most Memorable Dreams and Nightmares of Childhood*, from which many of the themes in this chapter are drawn.

Why does it matter that children learn from the earliest possible age to respect and pay close attention to their dreams? Because dreaming is a natural capacity of all humans that reflects our innate powers of creative imagination. Setting aside the meaning of individual dreams, the fact that humans have dreams *at all* indicates the deeply rooted nature of this aspect of brain–mind functioning. Thanks to these powers of creative imagination, humans have been able to explore, adapt, innovate, and grow in a wide variety of different environmental conditions. We are a dreaming species, and we can see the first emergence of this capacity in early years of childhood.

The prevalence of nightmares in childhood has many causes. Neglect, abuse, and trauma are unfortunately very consistent sources of recurrent nightmares. Frightening dreams are one of the most common reactions to traumatic experiences, and children can be especially vulnerable when a personal or collective disaster strikes. Parents, teachers, and others should be attentive to the occurrence of such nightmares when children go through traumatizing situations. The bad dreams can serve as a kind of emotional barometer to gauge the children's subjective experiences of the external threats.[3]

Yet, not all children's nightmares are caused by such problems. Some dreams of childhood are experienced as intensely frightening because they suddenly open up dramatic new dimensions of the unconscious mind, dimensions that seem completely alien to the waking self yet are filled with tremendous energy and emotion. The fear in the dream comes not from an external threat of violence, but from the startling power of a strong inner impulse toward growth and maturation. This is why children who have no unusual stress or trauma in their lives can still have recurrent nightmares. The dreams are pointing toward a future of psycho-spiritual development that will be difficult, frightening, and painful, but also tremendously joyful and fulfilling when the dangers are overcome and the new growth is achieved.

This chapter will outline an approach to the interpretation of children's nightmares drawing on Jung's theory and practice of dreams, along with current psychological research on dreaming. We will discuss three brief case studies to illustrate our approach and show how simple it is to apply in practice. This approach does not necessarily yield automatic answers or miracle healings, but it does help to open up the exploration of children's dreams in a way that can lead in any of several beneficial and insightful directions.

A Jungian Approach to Dream Analysis

Our approach is grounded in the work of Swiss psychologist C. G. Jung (1875–1961) and his theory of the dynamic relationship between the consciousness of each individual person and the collective unconscious shared by all humans. Jung took special interest in childhood nightmares as one of the best places to watch the emerging relationship between consciousness and the unconscious in a person's life. He referred to these kinds of vivid and highly memorable dream experiences from childhood as "big dreams" and he saw them as extremely valuable revelations of inner potential and future development in a child's life.[4] From a Jungian perspective, childhood nightmares offer a unique opportunity to witness the growth of the living psyche. This chapter will draw upon Jung's ideas to describe several practical principles to help in exploring and understanding the nightmares of childhood. Foremost among these methods is a playful engagement with the dramatic themes, characters, and settings of the dream.

As many but perhaps not all readers know, Jung was trained as a medical doctor and psychiatrist who originally worked in a clinic helping to heal people of their mental illnesses. In the early 1900s he formed a close friendship with Sigmund Freud, the Viennese psychiatrist whose book *The Interpretation of Dreams* was a landmark study of dreams as a means of exploring the unconscious depths of the human mind. Jung helped Freud develop the new model of psychoanalysis that emphasized the role of instinctual desires, early life experiences, and cultural influences in shaping an individual's personality.

The two men broke off their relationship in 1914, in part over their different ideas about dreams and the development of the mind. Jung was convinced that dreams were not merely the fulfillment of infantile wishes, as Freud claimed, but rather were natural expressions of the human psyche as it grew and processed experiences over time. These dream expressions might include infantile wishes, and they might include other things, too, like prospective anticipations of future possibility. Jung encouraged people to have an open mind about what might appear in dreams: "I proceed from the very simple principle that I understand nothing of the dream, do not know what it means, and do not conceive an idea of how the dream image is embedded in each person's mind."[5]

In practical terms, Jung advocated using a specific four-part template when trying to interpret a big dream from childhood. Jung taught the basic principles of using this template during a series of graduate school seminars he gave in Zurich from 1936 to 1940. A new translation of Jung's lectures and the class discussions appeared in 2008 in *Children's Dreams: Notes from the Seminar 1936–1940*. This book offers the best illustration yet of how Jung approached the challenge of interpreting early childhood dreams.

For the purposes of analysis and interpretation, Jung conceived of dreams as individual dramatic productions, like personalized plays. Using this metaphorical framework of a theatrical performance, Jung divided each dream into four elements:

1. Locale: The place and time of the dream and a list of the characters.
2. Exposition: The situation at the start of the dream, the beginning of the plot.
3. Peripeteia: How the plot develops, where it goes, what changes.
4. Lysis: The result, solution, closure; how it ends.

This method is not a magic formula that automatically determines the true meaning of the dream. On the contrary, it is a means of opening up the discussion and facilitating further exploration of where the possible meaning(s) of the dream may be found. Jung said that most big dreams have this basic narrative structure, so it helps to start the interpretive process by identifying those elements in the dream that correspond to this four-part dramatic schema. He acknowledged that not all dreams have a clear-cut lysis or conclusion, which can be a sign of an unresolved conflict.

Once these narrative features have been noted, the discussion turns to the potential role of the dream in the child's growth and development. In some cases the dream may reflect an obstacle or impediment to growth. In other cases the dream may reveal new powers and unexpected opportunities. The dreams can relate to unresolved conflicts from the past, difficult challenges in the present, and/or inspiring hopes for the future. There are many, many possible dimensions of meaning! The deepest meanings of any dream are ultimately rooted in the unique life circumstances of each individual. This is why any outside guidance, like the advice we are giving in this chapter, has to be balanced with your personal judgment and evaluation of the life context of the dreamer.

To help illustrate some of these ideas as they play out with an actual dream, we will draw on some of the examples we described in greater length in our *Children's Dreams* book from 2012. In that book we use Jung's four-part template to analyze and discuss several children's dreams we gathered from various sources. As we note there, we do not try to pursue every possible layer of meaning in the dreams. Instead, we limit ourselves to highlighting aspects of meaning that can be identified fairly easily and relate to collective human experience. Almost every dream has its own distinctive, idiosyncratic qualities that make it different from other dreams. This is why it is impossible to write a universal dictionary of dream symbols: the potential variations of dreaming experience are virtually infinite. That makes it more difficult to work with dreams, but it also testifies to the incredible creativity of the dreaming imagination.

Brenda's Dream

The first dream we will mention comes from a preschool child of about four years of age. Typically, the dreams of children in this age range (two to five years old) tend to be quite brief, with few characters and not much action. The characters are usually known to the dreamer (family or friends), and they include a higher frequency of animal characters than do the dreams of adults. The settings tend to be home or homelike, and the child watches what happens in the dream as a passive observer. According to empirical research by David Foulkes and others, these are the baseline features of "little" dreams in childhood. When a child of this age has a "big" dream, it often has many of these same features, but with greater intensification of imagery, feeling, and narrative engagement. The experience goes from being "just a dream" to something so impactful that it remains a vivid presence in the person's memory for the rest of their lives.

Brenda (not her real name) said she began having this recurrent dream when she was four, and she could still remember it several decades later when she was an adult:

> *My family (there were people with me and it had the feeling of my family although I never saw their faces) was at home (but it really was not our house in the dream.) The house was on fire. Flames were shooting up around things but not burning them. We had to exit the house from the upstairs. I had to leave my beloved stuffed bunny on the couch. I could have easily saved him but I did not. I was not afraid of the fire. It was upsetting to me to have to leave the bunny.*

We can start by determining which parts of Brenda's dream report fit into Jung's four-part template:

Locale:	A place that feels like home, but is not the physical structure where she and her family live. The time seems to be the present. The characters are a vague collection of her family and her stuffed bunny.
Exposition:	Her home is on fire.
Peripatea:	She and her family flee the fire.
Lysis:	She leaves her stuffed bunny behind.

The plot of the dream was brief, the setting homelike, and the characters familiar. In these ways it is a typical "little" dream from early childhood. Yet despite its simplicity, Brenda's dream made a powerful impact on her imagination. She could remember it very clearly more than 40 years later, when she told it to us. The recurrence of the dream certainly accounts for a large part of its memorability. When a dream comes more than once, it nearly always signals an urgent concern coming from the unconscious mind, a concern about something that holds special significance for the individual's waking life. Many of the nightmares of childhood are recurrent, with each new instance reinforcing the emotional impact of the underlying theme.

Brenda's dream starts with a strange ambiguity about her setting and companions. She is at home, but not exactly her current house. She is with her family, but she cannot see their faces. When dreams have vague uncertainties like this, it can indicate a shift in the individual's awareness to deeper unconscious realities, away from the ordinary concerns of daily life. Brenda's recurrent dreams were not just about her personal home and family; they were also about the collective human experience of homes and families.

That symbolic home is on fire. Fire is an important theme in children's dreams; here in Brenda's dream, fire is a source of danger and destruction. This might indicate emotional problems within her family, although Brenda said she had a good, nontraumatic childhood. The dream is silent about who or what set the fire. The flames just start, quickly consuming her home and threatening her family. Strangely, she says she has no fear of the fire. It endangers everything and everyone else, but she is not scared of it. What can account for that?

Perhaps because she knows at an unconscious level how quickly she is growing up. She knows she will survive the rising flames because they reflect her own rising development. The burning energy of fire is actually more than just a metaphor of growth. It literally expresses the accelerating chemical dynamics of that physical growth in the child's metabolism and neurological development. In this sense, her dream is a prospective vision of where that growth is leading her.

The odd detail about escaping the fire by going upstairs might be explained as a reference to "growing up." The fiery pace of Brenda's growth will eventually destroy her early childhood life as she rises up to become her future self.

An important feature of Brenda's recurrent dreams is that they concentrate her awareness not on where she is going, but on what she must leave behind, namely her stuffed bunny. As any parent knows, a child's stuffed animal can become the object of intense emotional attachment. Such beloved figures enable children to explore the complicated world of interpersonal relationships and try out various kinds of social behavior in a safe, emotionally manageable space. In Brenda's dreams her stuffed bunny seems to metaphorically represent her own early childhood, conveying a message that to grow up she must leave the bunny behind.

The bunny also embodies her emerging capacity to mourn, to accept experiences of loss, feelings of sadness, and the inevitability of change. Brenda could have gone back to save her bunny, but she chose not to do so. In that poignant moment, which her dreams repeated again and again for extra emotional emphasis, Brenda confronted a deep existential truth about human life: We cannot go back. To enter a new developmental stage is to leave an old stage behind. Brenda's dream prepared her for the impending loss of early childhood and taught her about the creative destruction at the fiery core of human growth.

The spiritual gift of this dream is a vision of transformation. Like an alchemical reaction, the magical fire changes one substance into another, creating something even more precious and valuable than before. That substance is Brenda's young psyche, emerging from the flames with new wisdom and maturity.

Hector's Dream

The second example comes from middle childhood, when school has become a regular part of children's lives and their social world has expanded beyond the immediate family to include a wider range of people. As research by David Foulkes (in his 2009 book *Children's Dreaming and the Development of Consciousness*) and other psychologists have shown, cognitive skills are also expanding rapidly at this age, with growing capacities for self-directed action and abstract mental processing. These changes have an impact on both the form and content of children's dreams, which typically become longer and more detailed, with greater physical activity, more narrative sophistication, and a wider range of settings and characters. There are more references to cultural themes from movies, books, and video games, and an expanded range of perspectives within the dreaming experience.

Hector (not his real name) was a nine-year-old boy who reported this dream in response to a question asking him about the most memorable dream he could ever remember:

> *I was riding my bike and it was a sunny day. Then it started raining with thunder and lightning. I had to walk my bike home because I couldn't ride it in the rain. I came home and my parents were sleeping in their bed. I went to my bedroom and saw myself sleeping in my bed. Then I was dreaming that I was sleeping. I left the room and the dream started all over again from riding my bike. I felt weird.*

Here is the four-part analysis of Hector's dream:

Locale:	The setting begins someplace outside near his home, then moves into the house. The characters are his parents and himself.
Exposition:	He is riding his bike on a sunny day.
Peripateia:	A storm hits and forces him to walk his bike back home. Inside he sees his parents asleep, and then he sees himself asleep and realizes he is dreaming.
Lysis:	He loops back to the beginning of the dream.

The opening of the dream sounds like an idyllic moment of middle childhood. Younger children generally cannot ride bikes by themselves, but school-aged children can, and Hector's dream starts with him enjoying the privileges of this age-appropriate ability: mobility, independence, speed. Riding a bicycle is a big developmental achievement in terms of the physical skills necessary for keeping your balance. To be able to ride a bike means that your body has gained a powerful new sense of orientation and control. There's a saying that once you learn to ride a bike, you never forget. It's a small but meaningful turning point from younger to middle childhood.

The sunny weather parallels the positive physical and psychological energy of his bike riding. Weather often appears in dreams as an aspect of outer nature (the environment, the elements) and also inner nature (emotions, the collective unconscious). In Hector's dream both dimensions seem to be in play. The sunny weather provides ideal environmental conditions and also mirrors the "sunny" enthusiasm that children generally experience cruising along on their bikes.

Then the weather changes, and Hector's dream takes a sharp turn in a darker direction. Humans instinctively react to sudden changes in the weather with alarm and wonder. When a storm suddenly hits it catches our attention, and we instantly shift into a threat-assessment mode of thought, trying to reorient in the new conditions and find a safe place to take shelter. A consequence of children getting old enough to set out on the road by themselves is that they become more vulnerable to such abrupt and dangerous shifts in the weather. What starts as a pleasantly sunny day suddenly turns into a raging thunderstorm. Here, Hector does not indicate any sense of personal danger from the storm, but he completely loses the power of riding his bicycle, and everything that goes with that. He has to use his feet again, and he has to go back home.

The primal forces of thunder, lightning, and rain have various symbolic shades of meaning and significance, not all of them negative. In Hector's dream the storm turns him away from a typical daytime activity and toward a realm of insight and knowledge that makes him feel "weird." The storm takes him out of a familiar setting and brings him to a place where his awareness shifts dramatically.

Ironically, this place of altered consciousness is his family home. Driven by the storm, Hector goes into the house and sees his parents asleep in bed. Freud would probably identify this image as a child's disguised fantasy of parental sexuality. That could be an accurate inference; most children by the age of nine have some idea about the birds and the bees, and it's natural for them to wonder what their parents do together in bed.

But the stronger emphasis of Hector's dream seems to be on the fact that his parents are sleeping, just as he finds himself sleeping a moment later. His parents are unconscious, while he is conscious. He is aware of them, but they are not aware of him. He comes home from the storm with a new perspective that transcends that of his parents. He knows things they do not know.

Then the dream takes an even more dizzying turn: He encounters himself, sleeping in his bedroom. At this point Hector realizes he is dreaming of sleeping. His perspective now transcends not only his parents, but his own physical body. This moment of lucid self-awareness leads him back to the beginning of the dream, which starts over again in what seems like a recurrent loop (perhaps linked symbolically to the endlessly round wheels of his bicycle). Hector's dream seems to have exposed him to a fundamental paradox of human consciousness: Once the process of self-reflection has begun, there is no end to the levels of awareness you may reach—and no way of knowing whether you are at the beginning or the end, the observer or the observed.

The third example comes from another nine-year-old boy, whose dream provides an early anticipation of puberty. The transition from middle childhood into adolescence and the teenage years is, of course, fraught with a host of developmental challenges, all of which are reflected in dreaming. This is the time when dream patterns begin to adopt the shape they will have in adulthood in terms of the kinds of characters, settings, themes, and interactions that are most frequent. But the whirlwind of developmental changes in physical, emotional, social, and intellectual aspects of life can spark extremely intense dreams that go far beyond the ordinary sphere of waking life, suggesting exciting but potentially dangerous directions for future growth.

William's Dream

William (not his real name) was a patient of one of the psychiatrists who attended Jung's seminars in 1936–1940. He told the dream during the course of therapy many years later:

> *I had a dream: From the street one could go down into a strange store. Richard and I went down. Three young women sat at a small table behind the counter. They gave us red sticks that we did not have to pay for: Like sealing-wax that one could smoke. So we put them into our mouths and started to smoke. Then I staggered out of the store; I'd gotten all dizzy and sick.*

Locale:	The setting is a strange subterranean store. The characters include a male friend and three young unfamiliar women.
Exposition:	He and his friend go down into the store.
Peripateia:	The three young women give them red sticks to smoke.
Lysis:	He leaves the store feeling disoriented and nauseous.

A male friend accompanies William, suggesting he is not the only person going through this process. They leave the ordinary daylight world of the street and go down into the ground, into an archetypal realm of mystery and magic. William calls it a "strange store," presumably meaning some kind of business where goods are kept, bought, and sold. As a symbol of the collective unconscious, the strange store is a place where William and his friend make contact with the archetypal powers of reproductive desire that will soon take on a driving importance in their waking lives.

These powers take the form of three young women, sitting at a table behind a counter. Their position indicates the store belongs to them. It is their place. They are the proprietors, the keepers of the goods, the arbiters of exchange. Jung and his students amplified this image of the three young women by referring to the three Fates of ancient Greek mythology (see Hamilton's 1942 *Mythology*), a group of shape-shifting, awe-inspiring women who guide the destiny of each human life. Jung also saw connections with the Holy Trinity of Christianity and the divine symbolism of the number three. We would add the three witches at the beginning of Shakespeare's play *Macbeth*, the "weird sisters" who accurately foretell Macbeth's future rise and fall.

The three women give William and his friend a very specific kind of object—red sticks made of sealing-wax. William may have had personal associations to the sealing-wax that could lead to other dimensions of meaning, but we can point out the ordinary function of sealing-wax as a means of closing a letter or other form of personal communication. This suggests the sticks are somehow a means of sending a private message from the women to the boys. Sealing-wax is also a substance that changes form when heated, echoing the theme of transformation, and the red color enhances the connection to fire, heat, and passion.

Unlike a normal store, no money is exchanged. The sticks are a gift from the three young women to William and his friend. The boys put this gift to their mouths and breathe in the smoke. No actual fire is mentioned, but the sticks function like cigarettes in transforming a substance outside the body into a substance that can travel inside the body. They complete the process of absorbing the women's gift into the boy's physical being.

In today's world many people may have negative associations with cigarette smoking, but in this dream the smoking seems to be symbolic of the changes these women are bringing into William's life. Jung said, "The boy is here being initiated, for the first time, into sexuality."[6]

The smoke knocks him off balance and shifts his perception in unexpected ways. William's ego in the dream experiences this as unpleasant and nauseating, but as Jung pointed out, "what is disgusting is the unacceptable 'other' "[7] that must be integrated into consciousness if a person is to develop a healthy and balanced personality. William returns to the level of the street a changed person, aware of feelings and sensations he never knew before.

Practical Advice

When children are in immediate distress, the best thing of course is to comfort and reassure them, usually with hugs, soothing words, and sympathetic listening. These are almost always the most effective things to do when children wake up from a nightmare—hold them close, let them know you are right there with them, and reassure them that the dream is over and they are awake now. Turning on the lights for a while, getting a glass of water, and checking the safety of the room (e.g., making sure that nothing is lurking under the bed or hiding in the closet) can provide additional methods for helping children calm down from the intense feelings of the nightmare and eventually get back to sleep.

Having said all that, our advice is that parents should try to resist the temptation to say "it was just a dream" as a way of reassuring their children in these situations. It may be well-meaning, but the phrase "just a dream" inevitably suggests that dreams are not "real," and thus not worthy of any special attention or concern. Dreams *are* real, however: real in their feelings and their perceptual sensations, and real in their potential significance for the dreamer's life. Dreams are different from waking reality, of course, but they have their own reality that should be acknowledged and respected. Telling children "it was just a dream" sends the wrong message: instead of taking dreams seriously, it dismisses them as irrelevant. As an alternative, a parent could say, "That was a scary dream, but it's over now, and you're awake and with me and with _____ (fill in the name of the child's favorite stuffed animal)." Parents can help their children make clear distinctions between waking and dreaming without demeaning the significance of the latter.

The Dream as a Lifelong Companion

As these examples indicate, the exploration of a big dream from childhood can lead in many different directions. There is no clear-cut destination, no final answer to these explorations. Rather, they offer an opportunity to expand one's awareness of oneself, family, community, and the world at large. Such dreams lead deep into the self, as a means of gaining new perspectives on external reality.

Over the course of a lifetime, the meanings and significance of early childhood nightmares can subtly change as additional layers of life experience reveal new dimensions previously unappreciated in the original dream. In this way the dream can become a kind of lifelong companion, guiding the dreamer along the path of *individuation*, which was Jung's term for the innate tendency toward a whole, balanced, and integrated personality. The basic idea here is that the psychological development of all humans follows a common instinctual template, inscribed in the structure of our minds and the coding of our genes, and taking a unique shape in the particular context of each individual's life. Big dreams are like guideposts in that developmental process, helping integrate the conscious and unconscious, the personal and collective, the light and the darkness within each of us.

This process is not necessarily "religious," although it often becomes intimately associated with a variety of religious images, symbols, and ritual practices. It could be called *spiritual*, although that term by itself might suggest something ethereal and disembodied, and big dreams are anything but that with their strong emotions, kinesthetic sensations, and physical carry-over effects (e.g., waking up sweating, breathing hard, startled, sexually aroused, etc.). In a book like this, with an audience of people from many different backgrounds, we prefer the term *psycho-spiritual* to indicate (a) the roots of big dreams in the psychological functioning of the brain–mind system as it has evolved over millions of years, and (b) the extension of big dreaming beyond basic psychological health (important as that is) to consider profound existential issues of truth, morality, death, the origins of the cosmos, and the nature of reality. When we speak in the title of childhood nightmares as a "gift," we mean a gift of psycho-spiritual value: something that connects children to the deepest sources of instinctual wisdom of the psyche and guides them in expressing that wisdom and developing their individuality in the unique circumstances of their embodied lives.

Notes

1. See, for example, Van de Castle, *Our Dreaming Mind*, and Young, *Dreaming in the Lotus*.

2. Including Hartmann, *The Nightmare*, and Revonsuo "The Reinterpretation of Dreams."

3. For more see Siegel and Bulkeley, *Dreamcatching*, especially Chapter 7, "First Aid for Crisis Dreams: Dream Patterns in Response to Crisis, Injury, Disability, Abuse, and Grief."

4. See Jung, "On the Nature of Dreams."

5. Jung, *Children's Dreams*, 23.

6. Ibid., 35.

7. Ibid., 39.

Bibliography

Bulkeley, Kelly and Patricia M. Bulkley. *Dreaming Beyond Death: A Guide to Pre-Death Dreams and Visions.* Boston, MA: Beacon Press, 2006.

Bulkeley, Kelly and Patricia M. Bulkley. *Children's Dreams: Understanding the Most Memorable Dreams and Nightmares of Childhood.* Lanham, MD: Rowman & Littlefield, 2012.

Foulkes, David. *Children's Dreams: Longitudinal Studies.* New York: Basic Books, 1982.

Foulkes, David. *Children's Dreams and the Development of Consciousness.* Cambridge, MA: Harvard University Press, 2009.

Freud, Sigmund. *The Interpretation of Dreams.* Translated by James Strachey. New York: Avon Books, 1965.

Hamilton, Edith. *Mythology: Timeless Tales of Gods and Heroes.* New York: Little, Brown and Company, 1942.

Hartmann, Ernest. *Nightmare: The Psychology and Biology of Terrifying Dreams.* New York: Basic Books, 1986.

Jung, C. G. "On the Nature of Dreams," in *Dreams.* Translated by R.F.C. Hull. Princeton, NJ: Princeton University Press, 1974, 67–84.

Jung, C. G. *Children's Dreams: Notes from the Seminar Given in 1936–1940.* Translated by Ernst Falzeder and Tony Woolfson. Princeton, NJ: Princeton University Press, 2008.

Revonsuo, Antii. "The Reinterpretation of Dreams: An Evolutionary Hypothesis of the Function of Dreaming," in *Sleep and Dreaming: Scientific Advances and Reconsiderations.* Edited by Edward Pace-Schott, Mark Solms, Mark Blagrove, and Stevan Harnad. Cambridge, UK: Cambridge University Press, 2003, 85–109.

Siegel, Alan and Kelly Bulkeley. *Dreamcatching: Every Parent's Guide to Exploring and Understanding Children's Dreams and Nightmares.* New York: Three Rivers Press, 1998.

Van de Castle, Robert. *Our Dreaming Mind.* New York: Ballantine, 1995.

Young, Serinity. *Dreaming in the Lotus: Buddhist Dream Narrative, Imagery, and Practice.* Somerville, MA: Wisdom Publications, 1995.

CHAPTER THREE

The Healing Power of Story: Re-Dreaming the Dream

Clare R. Johnson and Jean M. Campbell

I dreamed that a big tractor with heavy tires came right by, very close, and ran right over a baby tree.[1]

Mindy, age 5

The saying goes that "eyes are the window to the soul." The same thing can be said of dreams. Dreams reveal to us the state of our soul. They mirror our feelings and preoccupations by painting a cinematic picture of how we are experiencing life at that moment. Dreaming is a universal language, one which speaks in images, metaphors, and emotions that can be felt in the body. Story speaks the same language as dreams, which is why story carries a universal power—it draws on deep, collective imagery and passes messages through metaphor. Dreams and stories are woven from the same cloth, so story can be used as a healing art when working with dreams and nightmares.

Young children up to the age of around 10 do not always communicate as well through words as they can through images and stories, especially when talking about painful emotions. Children will tend to find it easier to talk about the dream they had of a dead witch rather than be asked outright: How do you feel about your mother leaving the family home? When children cannot express their feelings, sharing a dream and ultimately transforming it through storytelling can be instrumental in helping children to find the inner resources they need to tackle their current life situation. In this way, dreamplay—which can be defined as working and playing with a dream for therapy, empowerment, or fun—can lift children's deep unspoken concerns into consciousness without naming them directly.

Child psychotherapist and parenting expert Margot Sunderland notes: "children choose metaphor and story as their natural language for feeling, and do so because its indirect expression offers them protection ... all the healing work can happen entirely through your empathising *within the metaphor of the story*, so talking about real life is certainly not necessary for resolution and change."[2] This statement may sound surprising until we consider the exceptionally vivid reality of inner worlds such as dreams and the imagination. For children, inner worlds are extremely powerful, which is why when we speak to children through their own inner landscapes and imagery, we can reach them just as effectively—and often more effectively—than when we discuss life situations with them directly. We tend to place "real life" over and above every other reality, but how do we qualify "realness"? How real are dreams?

When I (Clare Johnson) was three years old, I dreamed that I was drowning in a turquoise swimming pool. With a flash of lucidity, I realized I could either stay in the dream and drown, or escape by waking myself up. I chose to wake up, throwing myself out of bed in the process. The crash alerted my mother, who came running. I told her, "I dreamt I was drowning!" Her response was to tell me that it was not real, it was just a dream.

Not real?

The colors and sensations of my dream were still utterly vivid in my mind. The experience seemed even more real than waking life. Just a dream? At that moment I began to grasp that there were two different worlds, both equally real, but for some strange reason only one of them counted. The dream world was silly; something meaningless that should be forgotten as soon as possible.

The dismissive "just a dream" response seems fairly standard when parents are faced with a distressed child following a nightmare. Although it is kindly meant, sadly it is unhelpful as the child does not feel heard or understood. Dreams, and especially nightmares, can form part of a child's long-term memories.[3] On an experiential level, *dreams are real*. Dreams are also stories: A dream can tell a complete story from opening scene to denouement, but it can also be an unfinished cliff-hanger or a broken story. Therefore, dreams can be seen as experientially real stories cocreated by the dreamer and the dreaming mind. Existing therapies such as Imagery Rehearsal Therapy[4] successfully use the "re-dreaming the dream" storytelling method with sufferers of post-traumatic stress disorder, while techniques such as Swiss psychiatrist Carl Jung's "Active Imagination" guide people to engage imaginatively with internal imagery to create psychological change. The effectiveness of these techniques indicates that dreams, stories, and the imagination can be combined in transformative and healing ways in the waking state.

In the first half of this chapter, I explore the healing power of story in young children aged 4–12 through an exploration of how nightmares can be transformed into empowering stories through lucid dreaming and its waking equivalent—my Lucid Storytelling Technique. In the second half of the chapter, Jean Campbell discusses the healing stories of teens and young adults.

From Nightmare to Empowering Story

Late one night, I found that Olivia (4) was still awake and moving her hands and feet back and forth rhythmically. I asked if she was cold, but she replied, "No, mommy. I'm trying to stay awake. If I don't sleep, I won't have a bad dream." The depth of her distress and anxiety over her recurring nightmares was brought to my full awareness at that moment. Her nightmares were on the verge of affecting her physical and mental health by keeping her awake at night.[5]

Nightmares are extremely common in young children. A study by Peter Muris et al. published in the *Journal of Clinical Child Psychology* found that 80 percent of school children aged 4–12 reported scary dreams. These were common in four- to six-year-olds and grew even more prominent in seven- to nine-year-olds, before decreasing from the age of ten.[6] Many parents feel helpless when faced with their child's nightmares. Particularly in the case of recurrent nightmares, parents feel they would do anything to make these "bad" dreams go away. But nightmares are not simply unwelcome events to be vanquished and eliminated: as Carl Jung pointed out, they can be powerful, creative, and healing gifts.[7]

Yet, try telling this to a parent whose child is waking up screaming every night. Some children become so fearful of their nightmares that they fight sleep with all their might. This creates an unbearable situation for children and parents alike and can spiral into bedtime disputes, sleep deprivation, daytime fatigue, and loss of concentration, all of which leads to more "bad" behavior until the evening rolls around and the whole exhausting battle begins again. This is not just the child being awkward. Nightmares feel utterly real: the child who dreams about a jaguar chasing and eating her can feel its claws ripping into her flesh. Yes, this experience happens in the dream state, so the child wakes up without a scratch on her body, but the psychological trauma of reliving such experiences can create long-lasting scars. The child takes matters into her own hands and decides that the world of sleep and dreams is not for her. Who can blame her? Who in their right mind would willingly enter a world where they know that dreadful things will happen to them? When nightmares become this strong, action must be taken because the child needs to be protected and empowered.

Lucid dreams are dreams where the dreamer is aware that he or she is dreaming. This conscious awareness can be used to guide and shape the dream if so desired. In my Deep Lucid Dreaming website interview series, I asked children's author Renée Frances how she helped her four-year-old to resolve the recurring nightmares that were making her scared of falling asleep.

> I really saw the lightbulb come on when I introduced Olivia to the idea of lucid dreaming. I told her that because the dreams are happening *in* her mind, rather than *to* her while she sleeps, *she* is the one who decides whom she meets and what kind of adventure she wants to have ... the power of storytelling as a key to helping with nightmares is *immeasurable*. Humans are inherently drawn to "the story."[8]

Lucid dreaming allows the dreamer to change the dream story while they are still in the dream. Renée Frances introduced her daughter to the concept of dreams as self-created, malleable stories. When the little girl understood that she could be an active participant in her own dream stories, she began to report happier dream scenarios such as making frightening dream bears go away. Thus empowered, she soon began to fall asleep within minutes of settling into bed. This heartening, transformative process became the inspiration for Frances's storybook *A Visit from the Good Night Fairy*.[9] For children who do not instantly master the art of lucid dreaming, my Lucid Storytelling Technique allows a similar transformative process to take place in the waking state.

Lucid Storytelling Technique: Empathize—Extend—Empower

When a child is helped to convert his nightmare into a waking version of a lucid dream, he can safely explore options for changing the dream story into something that makes him feel not terrified, but empowered. Adults can support children through empathizing, helping them to explore and extend their dream story, and empowering them to bring their new resources into their waking life.

Empathize

Give the child a safe space to talk through her nightmare. Borrowing her words and nightmare images, show the child you understand how the dream figures feel, but be careful of your own assumptions. Dream figures may represent an actual person in the child's life, an aspect of the child, or a particular emotion, so it is best not to assume the child identifies with the baby owl in the dream—she might identify more with the ogre! If you say, "The rabbit must feel lonely all on his own in the spaceship," the child may jump in and correct you if she feels you have got it wrong: "No, he's not lonely in the spaceship because all his friends live there." It is useful to take time to establish which dream figures and objects the child identifies with— is it the exploding volcano, the toilet paper, or the high-up eagle? Rather than making statements, try open questions such as: "I wonder how the eagle feels so high up in the sky?" When you understand more about the child's dream, you will know where and how to empathize. Empathizing shows the child that you have deeply heard her dream. It also helps you see how to guide her through the next step, that of extending the dream story.

Extend the dream story

The dreaming mind has already created the best possible metaphors for the child's feelings about his situation. Stay within the metaphors by continuing to speak in the language of the dream, and gently help the child to see the dream story as something that can be changed in any way they want to change it. However, all dreamplay should be child-led, which means respecting the child's decisions on what can and cannot be changed. If a child insists that there is no escape for the lamb stuck on a high ledge, there can be a temptation on the part of the adult to push for happier resolutions: "Surely if a rescue helicopter came along?" Yet for children it may be too early in the process, and they will either lose interest in this dream story which you, the adult, have swiped from their hands, or they will protest: "No! He can't ever get off the ledge!" Sometimes a child simply needs his "bad" feelings to be recognized and accepted by the adult[10] and so if a child is expressing through dream or metaphor that he feels lonely, stuck, and abandoned, he may not be ready to extend the dream story until he feels fully heard and understood.

Once the child seems ready, dreams and nightmares can be extended into stories with deeply satisfying outcomes for the child. The new dream story can help the child to see which behavioral patterns get good results and which do not. It can help children to find creative ways of responding to situations; first in their imagination, and later in waking life. It can develop their resourcefulness as they learn to find solutions and get help.

When she turned four, my daughter Yasmin started having nightmares after watching a "Dora the Explorer" episode where a bad witch disguises herself as a tree, then puts a little cartoon character under a spell. She started "seeing" bad witches in her bedroom in the dark. I responded by leaving the lights off and encouraging her to change what she saw: She turned the nastiest witch into a baby monkey and the others into flowers. Then we made up a story together about helping the baby monkey in the woods to find his mother so he would feel safe. After that, the nightmares never returned.

Here are some ideas for extending the dream story with children:

- Interview dream figures to find out what they are thinking and feeling. Ask them their motives: Why are you chasing me? What do you want?[11]
- If the child feels safe, he might want to try the Gestalt method,[12] where the dreamer imagines himself as different characters in the dream, slipping into their skin and speaking from their perspective. This method can work with dream animals, objects, even the dream sky, and can shed new light on the dream.
- Tell children about lucid dreaming and explain that if they know that they are dreaming, they can guide the dream. Ask children: What would you do if this were a lucid dream? Let them be as outrageous and imaginative as they like; let them blow off emotional steam making up exaggerated reactions to monsters if they want to. Imagining being lucid in the dream might be enough to create a satisfying story, but if need be you can help the child with specific questions such as:
- What does the dreamer need in this dream? Let the child give the answers: "She needs a pick axe to get out of the hole." "She needs a big dog to bark at the bad man and make him run away." Encourage the child to seek a solution to the dreamer's problem; then the child can test it by closing her eyes and re-dreaming the dream.
- Make sure children lead the story action—your job is to listen and offer possibilities if they get stuck, but the changed story and any solutions must be their own invention to have the power needed to resolve their nightmare.

Empower the child

In *Using Storytelling as a Therapeutic Tool with Children*, psychotherapist Dr. Margot Sunderland gives many striking examples of how creating dreamlike stories relying on archetypes and symbolism can help children suffering from trauma to recognize and change destructive behavioral patterns, and learn new coping strategies. She remarks: "Children often need to rehearse a different way of being (e.g., a softer, more gentle self, or a stronger, more assertive self) in fantasy via story, many times, before taking it into reality."[13] Let's consider five-year-old Mindy's dream at the start of this chapter for an example of how a child can begin to practice self-empowerment through re-dreaming the dream.

Ann Sayre Wiseman, author of *The Nightmare Solution*, worked on Mindy's dream of a baby tree being run over by a tractor by first asking her to draw it, and then asking her to speak in the voice of the tractor and the baby tree. Mindy was asked to create a solution to protect the baby tree: She drew a house around it, with a skylight in the roof so sunlight could shine through. Mindy closed her eyes to reenter the dream and see how the new dream story worked out. After reporting that the tractor had respected the protective house and had not run into it, she (unprompted) made a bridge to her waking feelings: "Sometimes I feel just like that little tree." Wiseman empathized: "It sounds like you know how it feels to be nearly mowed down." She then encouraged Mindy to empower herself by speaking of her feelings the next time she felt "mowed down": "Maybe in your waking life you could use the tree's message as a signal to speak up and remind people that you have feelings, too."[14]

- A sense of empowerment and satisfaction often comes when the children decide how they can help their dreaming selves. This might involve turning the dream into a funny story, summoning a friend, parent, or superhero to help, or using a magical object such as a wishing ring or an invisibility cloak to change events or create new escape routes.
- At the end of the storytelling process, sum up the dream story and check in with the child on how the main figure feels now.
- If it seems appropriate, a direct bridge may be made to the child's waking life situation, but this should not be forced by the adult as it may leave the child (who has been expressing herself indirectly through metaphor and symbolic language) feeling exposed or shamed. It can be just as effective to stay within the metaphor when summing up anything useful learned in re-dreaming the dream.

Storytelling can help children to reconfigure nightmares into empowering scenarios, creating strategies to help them access their inner resources. One five-year-old girl, Molly, dreamed she was at home alone and the house caught fire with her inside it. When she drew the dream and looked for solutions, it became clear that the reason she had not left the burning house in her dream was because she was under strict orders from her mother to stay put while her mother popped out to the store. The practical lesson this little girl needed to learn was that in emergency situations she could break parental rules and think for herself. In the story-picture, she added a policeman to help her cross the street so that she could find her mother and tell her to call the fire brigade. In her waking life, telling her mother about the dream prompted her mother to go through a fire drill with her so that Molly would feel empowered to know what to do if ever a fire happened when she was home alone.[15]

Re-dreaming the dream by day allows children to see much more clearly their emotions, reactions, and behavioral patterns, along with the motives

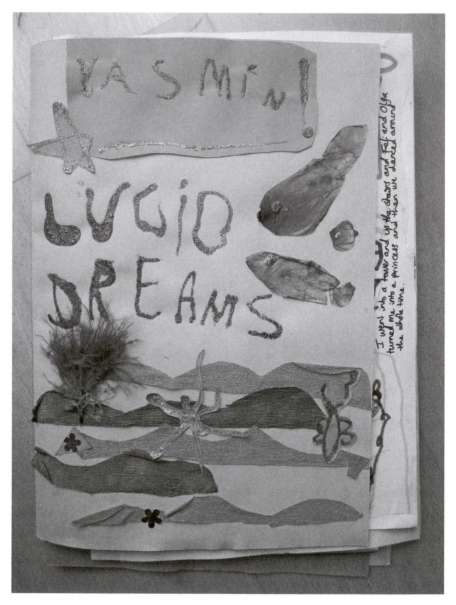

Figure 3.1   Lucid Dream Book (Yasmin Johnson, age 4)

of the people in their lives. When a child is encouraged to take charge and help her dreaming self, she learns valuable coping skills and resourcefulness, as well as potentially changing a pattern of helplessness or fear. Creating a book of dream art and dream stories can be done at any age, and this too can be empowering. Aged four, my daughter decided to make a "lucid dream book" and set about drawing and collaging her favorite lucid dreams using watercolors, glitter glue, dried petals, wool, and colored pens, as can be seen in Figure 3.1.

A study titled "Lucid dreaming in children: The UK library study," showed that the incidence of lucid dreams was most strongly associated with children who had a preference for reading science fiction and fantasy.[16] Habitually entering imaginal worlds while awake through the experience of reading fantasy stories could equip children with a greater ease in guiding the storytelling landscape of their dreams. Re-dreaming the dream teaches children that they can change terrifying nightmares into new stories. This lucid awareness of their ability to change things can carry over into children's waking lives, ultimately helping them to change their reactions to difficult life situations, heal past wounds, and become empowered.

Empowering Adolescents with Dream Story

As young people move into adolescence they often appear to have left the softness of dreams and childhood behind them. Being cool, being part of the peer group, opposing adult authority whether in school or out, are all part of the maturation process. Yet, as I (Jean Campbell) learned from years of teaching writing classes to teenagers, it is essential, sometimes lifesaving, for adults to remember that these adolescents are still children, looking for ways to grow safely into adulthood.

This principle was amply illustrated when, in the first writing class I taught to senior high school students, the year began with the assignment of writing a children's story. In preparation for the assignment, I told students I was going to read a story to them—in this case Seymour Leichman's delightful book *The Boy Who Could Sing Pictures*,[17] though there are many other books that can be used—for example, the ever-popular book about dreams by Maurice Sendak, *Where the Wild Things Are*.[18]

Having announced to the class that I would read to them, I looked up to find students standing up, moving their chairs. "What are you doing?" I asked feeling a little alarmed.

"We're putting our chairs in a circle so you can read to us," they replied. And for two classroom hours, like many groups to follow, they sat in a circle, as entranced by the story as any younger group might be.

This first writing assignment involving children's dreams begins: Write down a dream. The dream can be a recent one; an old one; or, if you do not remember your dreams, make one up. Then we will write some stories.

Assuming, with teenagers, that there will be a first round of giggling at this assignment, and recognizing that there will be some number of

"The Pizza That Ate New York" dreams invented by students, are both good assumptions for the writing teacher. But asking students to focus on a dream of their own generally produces a depth of experience that is not often seen in the classroom.

Perhaps you will be as fortunate as I was. When the time came for dreams to be read aloud to the group, several members of the football team, who had enrolled in the class as an easy elective, began to guffaw. They laughed until a pretty, blond cheerleader read her dream about talking with her recently deceased grandmother. The pair talked together in the family's horse barn where they often met in a dream state.

"You don't believe dreams are real?" she asked the somewhat shamefaced boys. "I meet my grandma in dreams a lot, and talking to her helps me to understand things."

Teenagers have a lot of questions about dreams: Are they "real"? If I die in a dream will I be dead? What happens if I fall off a tall building and hit the ground? What does it mean if I'm naked in a dream? What does it mean if I dream that I've missed a big exam? Can people really fly or be lucid in dreams? These are only some of the many questions that will come to the surface, if allowed.

Although it is not the role of the writing teacher to interpret dreams or discuss dreaming techniques, if one is going to bring up the subject of dreams, it helps to be prepared with at least some personal answers to these types of questions. Do not be afraid to answer dream questions with, "I don't know," or to tell students that they might want to begin keeping a dream journal to learn more about what they are dreaming. Dreams are uniquely individual. Reminding students that the best person to interpret the meaning of the dream is the dreamer also helps maintain a classroom balance; and telling students that dream dictionaries, by and large, though they may be useful to understanding cosmologies, are not much use in interpreting dreams, can be helpful as well.

For the teacher who is willing to allow for the opportunity of discussion, dreams can produce the ideal writing environment. People tend to be at their most creative when fully engaged with their subject, rather than simply performing a writing assignment. Writing from dreams allows that type of engagement.

Why Make Up a Dream?

Always give teens an out. Providing a space in which there is no need for young people to be embarrassed in front of their peers is an important aspect of any subject in any classroom. Many young people have low dream recall because they have never been encouraged to write down or pay attention to their dreams. In fact, the opposite may have been true. Students may have been told their dreams were insignificant or "just a dream."

But there are many aspects of dream awareness to be explored. Try asking students to write down how they feel when they first wake up. Did they remember a color or a sound? That, too, is information from the dreaming self. And what about The Voice? Often people will wake with only a word or a sentence, seemingly spoken by an unseen or disembodied voice. This is part of dreaming, too. For example, shortly after I began teaching, a pale, young teenager crept into my classroom before the day's classes began. I knew her to be troubled by the breakup of her parents' marriage and her need to care for younger siblings, while also holding down an after-school job. This is true today for many teens. "God spoke to me for the third time last night," she whispered to me almost inaudibly, bending over me where I sat at my desk.

Resisting the urge to ask what God had said the first two times He spoke to her, I asked, "What did God say?"

He said: "You've done good!" the girl replied, her face breaking into a smile. "He told me I've done good."

Although a primary value of dreams to storytelling comes from the fact that dreams often follow a recognizable story line, with introduction, denouement, and conclusion, thus allowing the teacher an opportunity to develop concepts of story construction, understanding that the dream state holds many aspects that cannot be identified as traditional story is an important way to delve into a dream story as well.

Writing for Quality: School Assignments

For the language or writing teacher, dreams provide an endless opportunity to explore terms students are required to know. Dreams are often couched in metaphor. For example, classic dreams such as forgetting to attend an exam or finding oneself in school naked are metaphors for the self-consciousness embarrassment so many teens feel. In dreams, objects such as an engagement ring or a football can be used to symbolize feelings about love and marriage, or (in the case of the football) feelings about playing sports or being one of a crowd.

Many people also dream in puns; and many dreams are a play on words, like the student who said he dreamed he was a lion and other students quipped: "Yes, he's always lion around!" or "He's been doing some lion, too!"

Students are often astonished to discover how many of the famous authors they are assigned to read in school: poets, filmmakers, novelists, storytellers, have drawn their works from dreams. Author Naomi Epel interviewed over 30 contemporary writers and artists for her book *Writers Dreaming*, asking them how they use dreams in their work. She quotes Poet Laureate Maya Angelou as saying: "Maybe a writer is hesitant to get to a depth in a character, to admit that this fictional character does this or thinks this or has acted this way—or that an event was really this terrifying—the brain says, 'Okay, you go on and go to sleep. I'll take care of it. I'll show you where that is.'"[19]

Author Stephen King when interviewed, talked about the writing process:

> Part of my function as a writer is to dream awake. And that usually happens. If I sit down to write in the morning, in the beginning of that writing session and the ending of that session, I'm aware that I'm writing. I'm aware of my surroundings. It's like shallow sleep on both ends, when you go to bed and when you wake up. But in the middle, the world is gone and I'm able to see better. Creative imaging and dreaming are just so similar that they've got to be related.[20]

Many of the classic authors assigned to students in classrooms have also, like more current authors, drawn upon their dreams for creative work: Samuel Taylor Coleridge, Mary Shelly, Mark Twain, Herman Hesse, Robert Louis Stevenson, and J. R. R. Tolkien, to name just a few. Understanding that these famous writers have also utilized dreams for creative purposes helps young writers to identify with what they are reading, and to understand how they too might function as writers.

As I point out in my book *Dreams Beyond Dreaming*[21] these first writing class assignments yielded interesting results at the academic level as well, even among students who were considered academically average or below. In the first year of the creative writing class described earlier, one of the dream-based short stories won first place in the State Writing Competition for students. Two years later, two young poets, both of them making average grades in their literature classes, won first and third prizes in the State Writing Competition for their poetry, written from dreams.

What Do Teens Dream?

As dream researcher Patricia Garfield points out to teenagers in her award-winning book *The Dream Book: A Young Person's Guide to Understanding Dreams*, as children begin to mature into teenagers:

> Your dreams are changing big-time. Those hormones you hear so much about not only cause guys to get beards and girls to get curvier bodies, but they can also create chaos in your dream life. Researchers tell us that the

quality of dreams changes as adolescence begins. Nice dreams decrease. Wild and wacky dreams increase. If you start having some crazy dream adventures, you should know that so does almost every other kid your age.

During the years you are doing the most growing, you are also dreaming more. The more you sleep, the more you dream. Soon you'll want to sleep more than you used to—you might have already noticed that you get drowsy more often. The same hormones that cause the radical changes in your body during adolescence also make you feel more sleepy than at any other time in your adult life (except during pregnancy for women).[22]

Although there are still relatively few studies done with children or teenage dreamers, due to the comparative difficulty involved with obtaining permissions from this age group, recent content-analysis research on a group of 102 reports of recurrent dreams in teenagers between 11 and 15, done by Aline Gauchat, Antonio Zadra, and others in the Psychology Department at the University of Montreal, indicates significant differences in the content of recurrent dreams of teenagers of those from adults. As the study points out, the most frequently reported, recurring dreams for this age group involved confrontations with monsters or animals, followed by physical aggressions, falling, and being chased. Recurrent dreams from this group were more likely to include negative content elements than positive ones.[23] All of these dream themes are common for children and teens as they make their way toward adulthood.

Because many adolescents appear to be so grown up, both physically and psychologically, it is sometimes easy for adults working with teenagers to forget they are still dealing with children. This can be detrimental to both the young person and the adult involved. Dream stories give us such insight into the lives of teens, particularly in cases where trauma or abuse is involved, that it is difficult to resist interpretation or action.

In these cases, it is essential to proceed with utmost care, remembering that in most areas of the world children are considered minors until they have reached the age of 18. They are, quite literally, in the custody of their parents, relatives, or in some cases the courts. Thus, any action taken toward providing assistance for teens must equally involve those adults in charge—no matter how mature the young person may appear.

The Added Value of Turning Dreams into Story

For teenagers, as well as for all children, the opportunity to explore dreams as story offers the additional value of time to discuss what is troubling them. Since dream characters often arise from the depth of intense concentration, even the simple exercise of writing a description of a dream character or dream episode for a writing class can be highly charged. And the ensuing conversation can help young people process deep feelings.

One example of this came when I asked a group of students to take a scene from a dream and describe it in writing as if it were a scene from a story. When these brief scenarios were read, one boy described himself as the dream character. He was bouncing a basketball against the sidewalk on the deserted streets of his neighborhood. In the dream, he was the only person left alive after a nuclear holocaust. This type of dream is far more common in the lives of teenagers than many might believe, as these young people face growing up in an uncertain world.

Immediately, when the well-written essay above was read, the room erupted into conversation. There was no need to encourage discussion as students revealed their own end-of-the-world dreams and fears of nuclear disaster. For all of them, because the conversation took place in the safety of a classroom, there was a depth of connection involved which would probably not be achieved in other activities—in or out of the classroom.

I hope you will be lucky enough to have the type of experience with teens working through their issues that I had one day when I asked a group of writing students to break into groups of six and develop the description of a dream character by having each person in the circle add a line of description after the dreamer wrote the initial, descriptive line. Students like this kind of sharing, which often produces interesting results and insights. I might have had more forethought than to allow six teenage boys with high IQs and creative minds to sit together for this exercise. But they were well-behaved and clearly working despite bursts of laughter, so I left them and the rest of the class to write their dream character descriptions, with time for reading them aloud before the end of the period.

One of the characters dreamed up by this group of boys was a young boy their age by the name of Joe Fredd. Among other things we learned about Joe Fredd was the fact that he was about to enlist in the Army, and was not feeling very comfortable about it. Like many of my students, Joe Fredd was facing career choices that would affect the course of his life. What happened next though was an unexpected explosion of creativity, as Joe Fredd burst from the classroom. At the end of the week, as I paused in the teacher's lounge to collect a book, another faculty member said to me: "Do you know a student by the name of Joe Fredd?"

What an innocent question. Alarm bells went off in my head. "Why?" I asked. Seems that Joe Fredd had come late to this teacher's class and turned in a hall pass. Only at the end of a busy class did the teacher realize he had no student by the name of Joe Fredd.

Cheering the creativity of my students, I kept quiet about the probable identity of Joe Fredd, but by the next week I had to confess my involvement. Joe Fredd had taken a test in Math class and done very well on it—except that the teacher was wondering who this invisible student might be. Since both Joe Fredd and his creator passed the test with flying colors, no more was said and nobody got in trouble. Pranks tapered off as graduation neared.

Joe Fredd continued to appear in my life however, as I received a continuing stream of "letters from Joe Fredd," when both he and his dream-loving creator shipped out for military training. Joe Fredd described the people he met on base, the instructors, how he felt about basic training. I am certain that, for the author, this alter ego provided a bit of relief from the hardships of a new life. For the younger students he'd left behind, including some of the original Joe Fredd conspiracy, the letters I read to them were an inspiration to greater writing adventures.

Not all dream-into-story results will be as dramatic as those described in this chapter, but for pure engagement of student attention there is no better basis than their own, nightly adventures. Dreams lead the way toward an exploration of feelings and creative ideas that can be infinitely useful and even world changing.

Notes

1. Ann Sayre Wiseman, *The Nightmare Solution* (USA, Echo Point Books, 2013), 82.

2. Margot Sunderland, *Using Storytelling as a Therapeutic Tool with Children* (London, Speechmark Publishing, 2000), 85.

3. Stephen LaBerge and Donald DeGracia, "Varieties of Lucid Dreaming Experience," in *Individual Differences in Cognitive Experience*, eds. Robert Kunzendorf and Benjamin Wallace (Amsterdam, John Benjamins, 2000), 269–307.

4. Barry Krakow, R. Kellner, D. Pathak, L. Lambert, "Imagery Rehearsal Treatment for Chronic Nightmares," *Behaviour Research and Therapy* 33, no. 7 (1995): 837–843.

5. Clare R. Johnson, "Deep Lucid Dreaming Interview Series with Renée Frances: How to Empower Children through Lucid Dreaming," http://deeplucid dreaming.com/2015/07/empower-children-lucid-dreaming/.

6. Peter Muris, Harald Merckelbach, Björn Gadet, and Vénique Moulaert, "Fears, Worries, and Scary Dreams in 4- to 12-year-old Children: Their Content, Developmental Pattern, and Origins," *Journal of Clinical Child Psychology* 29, no. 1 (2000): 43–52.

7. Carl G. Jung, *Memories, Dreams, Reflections*, ed. Aniela Jaffé (London, Collins and Routledge & Kegan Paul, 1963).

8. Deep Lucid Dreaming: http://deepluciddreaming.com/2015/07/empower-children-lucid-dreaming/.

9. Renée Frances, A Visit from the Good Night Fairy (Victoria, Canada, Friesen Press, 2014).

10. Sunderland, *Storytelling as a Therapeutic Tool*.

11. Paul Tholey and Kaleb Utecht, *Schöpferisch Träumen: Der Klartraum als Lebenshilfe* (Frankfurt, Klotz [1995] 2008).

12. Fritz Perls, *Gestalt Therapy Verbatim* (Gouldsboro, The Gestalt Journal Press [1969] 1992).

13. Sunderland, *Storytelling as a Therapeutic Tool*, 80.

14. Wiseman, *The Nightmare Solution*, 83.

15. Ibid., 86–89.

16. Michael Schredl, Josie Henley-Einion, Mark Blagrove, "Lucid dreaming in children: The UK library study," *International Journal of Sleep Research* 5, no. 1 (2012): 9498.

17. Seymour Leichman, *The Boy Who Could Sing Pictures* (New York: Doubleday & Co, 1968).

18. Maurice Sendak, *Where the Wild Things Are* (New York: Harper Collins, 1963).

19. Naomi Epel, *Writers Dreaming* (New York: Carol Southern Books, 1993), 30.

20. Ibid., 141.

21. Jean Campbell, *Dreams Beyond Dreaming* (Norfolk, VA: Donning Company Publishers, 1980), 90.

22. Patricia Garfield, *The Dream Book: A Young Person's Guide to Understanding Dreams* (New York: Tundra Books, 2002), 2.

23. Aline Gauchat, J. R. Seguin, E. McSween-Cadieux, and A. Zadra, "The Content of Recurrent Dreams in Young Adolescents," *Consciousness and Cognition* 37 (2015): 103111.

Bibliography

Campbell, Jean. *Dreams beyond Dreaming*. Norfolk, VA: Donning Company Publishers, 1980.

Epel, Naomi. *Writers Dreaming*. New York: Carol Southern Books, 1993.

Frances, Renée. *A Visit from the Good Night Fairy*. Victoria, BC: Friesen Press, 2014.

Garfield, Patricia. *The Dream Book: A Young Person's Guide to Understanding Dreams*. New York: Tundra Books, 2002.

Gauchet, A., J. R. Seguin, E. McSween-Cadieux, and A. Zadra. "The Content of Recurrent Dreams in Young Adolescents." *Consciousness and Cognition* 37 (2015): 103–111.

Johnson, Clare R. "Deep Lucid Dreaming Interview Series with Renée Frances: How to Empower Children through Lucid Dreaming." http://deeplucid dreaming.com/2015/07/empower-children-lucid-dreaming/.

Jung, Carl G. *Memories, Dreams, Reflections*. Ed. A. Jaffé, London: Collins and Routledge & Kegan Paul, 1963.

Krakow, B., R. Kellner, D. Pathak, L. Lambert, "Imagery Rehearsal Treatment for Chronic Nightmares." *Behaviour Research and Therapy* 33, no. 7 (1995): 837–843.

LaBerge, Stephen, and Donald DeGracia. "Varieties of Lucid Dreaming Experience," in *Individual Differences in Cognitive Experience*, eds. Robert Kunzendorf and Benjamin Wallace. Amsterdam: John Benjamins, 2000, 269–307.

Leichman, Seymour. *The Boy Who Could Sing Pictures*. New York: Doubleday & Co, 1968.

Muris, P., H. Merckelbach, B. Gadet, V. Moulaert, "Fears, Worries, and Scary Dreams in 4- to 12-Year-Old Children: Their Content, Developmental Pattern, and Origins." *Journal of Clinical Child Psychology* 29, no. 1 (2000): 43–52.

Perls, Fritz. *Gestalt Therapy Verbatim*. Gouldsboro, ME: The Gestalt Journal Press, [1969] 1992.

Schredl, Michael, Josie Henley-Einion, Mark Blagrove. "Lucid dreaming in children: The UK library study." *International Journal of Sleep Research* 5, no. 1 (2012).

Sendak, Maurice. *Where the Wild Things Are*. New York: Harper Collins, 1963.

Sunderland, Margot. *Using Storytelling as a Therapeutic Tool with Children*. London: Speechmark Publishing, 2000.

Tholey, Paul and Kaleb Utecht. *Schöpferisch Träumen: Der Klartraum als Lebenshilfe*. Frankfurt: Klotz, [1995] 2008.

Wiseman, Ann Sayre. *The Nightmare Solution*. Brattleboro, VT: Echo Point Books, 2013.

CHAPTER FOUR

Dreamplay for Children Facing Illness, Injury, and Physical Handicaps

Tallulah Lyons

I'm in a little boat. I fall into the big ocean. He's after me—the big shark with long, sharp teeth is eating me! Make him go away! I'm scared. Make him go away.

Miguel, age 8

When a child is ill, injured, or living with a physical handicap, dreams are a metaphoric mirror of the pain, physiological imbalances, and emotional disruptions that eradicate a sense of safety and well-being. Common dream themes include being attacked by insects or ravaging animals; being chased and attacked by menacing monsters; being smothered, restrained, confined, stabbed, dismembered. There are dreams of burning and drowning, dreams of being totally alone and helpless, dreams of objects or buildings exploding and crashing down. When a child is physically distressed, dreams also bring comfort and strength. Along with nightmares, dreams bubble up and evoke a sense of healing—a sense that everything is all right no matter the pain and anxiety of the situation.

Nightmares seem to predominate during times of particular crisis, including the onset of illness, before visits to doctors and unfamiliar procedures, before and after surgery, at times of high fever or extreme changes in the body. For children who have been hospitalized or homebound, nightmares also increase when it is time to return to school. This is especially true if illness has caused change in physical appearance (loss of hair or limbs) or if the child is unable to participate in normally expected ways (special needs such as diet, or time out to take medication or injections, or the need for a wheelchair).

Trembling and slapping her own tiny body, two-year-old Annie screams, "Ants, ants," as her temperature climbs to 104 degrees. "Mean dog, mean dog," sobs six-year-old Sam who wakes from a nightmare grasping his infected ankle. "I can't breathe. Get him off me!" moans fourteen-year-old Edwardo when waking in the middle of a full-blown asthma attack. He is dreaming again of a huge bony hand covering his nose and mouth. "A tidal wave—overwhelming—awful. I see it coming. I can't run." This is the recurring dream of Martha, age seventeen. The nightmare began when she was confined to a wheelchair at age twelve.

Just as dreams reflect the physical and emotional disruptions of illness, they can also bring powerful healing experiences with imagery and energy to help transform relationships to medical situations and to move through crisis with a felt sense of empowerment and support.

For 20 years, I have facilitated dream groups with adults facing cancer. I have identified several types of dreams that bring a sense of healing, a sense of renewal and hope, a sense of at-oneness and wholeness. Participants in my dream groups have reported many dreams in which they encounter a transformative numinous figure or object. Simply being in the presence of this "transcendent presence" evokes a sense of healing. Dream group members have also reported many dreams that renew resolution and bring guidance for moving through the cancer journey. Some healing dreams are spontaneous, but many arise in "waking dreams" during reflective and meditative work with nightmares. Slowly the imagery and energy of a disturbing dream transforms. Some of the transformed nightmares have been reminders of old traumas in which the dreamer found creative inner survival skills. It is as if some dreams want the dreamer to reclaim inner strengths that were helpful in the past. Occasionally, there have been healing dreams that correspond with actual remission of the cancer. These transformative dreams and healing journeys are explored in my book, *Dreams and Guided Imagery*.[1]

In recent interviews with parents, children, and pediatric health care professionals, I have found similar healing themes in the dreams of children who face serious illnesses, injury, or physical handicaps. In this chapter, I will provide examples and elaborate on the healing themes. I will share practical techniques for engaging with dreams through creative imagination. Names and identifying characteristics of children and families and the details of their stories and dreams have been changed to protect their privacy.

Dream Encounters with Divine Beings, Animal Guides, and Superheroes

Young children easily access the realm of numinous energies where they encounter highly charged beings and objects that evoke awe, wonder, and a sense of infinite possibility. Swiss psychologist C. G. Jung wrote in his *Collective Works* that the essence of healing experience resides in such encounters.[2] When a young child is physically distressed, divine beings, animal guides, and magical superheroes bring comfort, support, companionship, and courage.

Angels and Monsters: A Child's Eye View of Cancer is a beautiful book offered by the American Cancer Society that confirms the frequent presence of helpful supporters. Over a period of eight years, art therapist Lisa Murray conducted an expressive arts project with twenty-five children. Billy Howard, who photographed the children and their work, wrote in the introduction, "Many have found a path through imagination—to a wisdom that confronts our greatest fears with charity, humor, and affection."[3] In *Angels and Monsters*, the images of helpful allies range from magical animals like unicorns and talking dogs, to superheroes like Chemo Kid, guardian angels, and helpful monsters. Yes, helpful monsters. For one five-year-old, the fierce Godzilla used his power to rain down fire upon the cancer hospital.

Young children often make little or no distinction between waking and sleeping encounters with numinous beings. When relating their children's dreams, several parents commented that their child seemed certain the event actually happened. For example, Dory, age four, was hospitalized for a severe strep infection. Since her mother needed to be at home with younger siblings, her father stayed by her bedside. During the night Dory woke screaming, "Jesus is here!" The next morning she told her parents, "Daddy doesn't have to stay here tonight. Jesus came and he'll come back to stay with me again." She was very happy in spite of fever and pain.

Dreams of Becoming Brave, Confident, and Resilient

When parents or guardians have to dispense medicine or take a child to a traumatic medical appointment, many automatically implore, "Be brave." After the ordeal, an automatic response is, "Oh, you were so brave!" In interviews, several parents commented that one of the positive outcomes of living with chronic illness was their child's growing self-perception of being a tough, brave, and strong person. Dreams in which a child feels brave or acts with courage seem to restore a sense of well-being and bolster a sense of being in control.

A friend offered a poignant example. When Amy was a preteen, she was plagued with multiple allergies and was taken for frequent testing. During that time, she had a recurring dream she called, "The Man in the Attic." The man in the attic looked like a dirty, unkempt ragamuffin. Only Amy knew of his existence, and though he was scary, he also evoked a lot of curiosity. In each dream, Amy would garner courage to climb a hidden ladder that led from her bedroom to the attic. In dream after dream, she sneaked food from the kitchen and took it to the scruffy man so he would have strength to free himself from the attic. Each time, Amy woke from her dream with a proud sense of accomplishment. As an adult looking back on these vivid dreams, Amy surmised that the dreams were a reflection and affirmation of her growing courage to take charge of her fear, not only about the allergy treatments, but also other normal preteen stresses.

Dreams of Transcending Physical Limitations

Whether a child has cancer and loses hair in treatment, or is injured and loses a limb in surgery, or has cerebral palsy and no control over body movements, or simply a stomach virus and is bedridden for a day—any sick child suffers the stresses of physical limitation. Often nightmares reflect limiting conditions in dreams of being trapped, unable to move, run, see, or scream. Such nightmares carry feelings of extreme vulnerability and fear.

Sick, injured, or handicapped children also have dreams about overcoming or transcending physical limitations. Such dreams evoke healing feelings of freedom and joy and can help galvanize a sense of being who one wants to be no matter the limiting circumstances of the physical condition.

Randy was an avid soccer player when at age 13, he broke his leg in two places during the first game of the season. His leg was in a cast for several months and during that time, he dreamed of spreading his arms and soaring over a game in his soccer uniform to deliver power drinks to his team. The dream experience seemed to help turn the tide of deep disappointment. Randy remembers that after the dream, he felt more determination and confidence for facing the reality of his enforced limitations. Dreams of flying are commonly reported, and can provide exhilarating experiences for any child.

Another common healing dream is the dream of breathing underwater. Katie was 15 when she had her colon removed. After surgery, she dreamed of being out on a raft at the beach with friends. Suddenly, a big wave upended the raft and Katie felt herself struggling to fight back to the surface. Just as she thought her lungs would burst, Katie relaxed and took a deep breath. At that point, she realized she was breathing underwater. After her dream, Katie's feeling was one of gratitude for exceeding expected possibilities. The dream became a touchstone whenever she found herself getting depressed about her limitations. Dream expert Jeremy Taylor writes that when one dreams about breathing underwater, it is a highly significant metaphor for the dreamer's evolving strengths and awareness.[4]

Even children who suffer severe sensory deprivation can have dreams that take them beyond their limitations into the healing realm of joy. In a paper, "Dreams of the Blind," written for publication in the online journal, *Electric Dreams*, Richard Catlett Wilkerson reports on the work of several researchers.[5] One researcher, Joseph Jastrow, cites several dreams from Helen Keller who was both deaf and blind. In a letter to Jastrow, Keller wrote:

> *One night I dreamed that I was in a lovely mansion, all built of leaves and flowers. My thoughts declared the floor was of green twigs, and the ceiling of pink and white roses. The walls were of roses, pinks, hyacinths, and many other flowers, loosely arranged so as to make the whole structure wavy and graceful. Here and there I saw an opening between the leaves, which admitted the purest air. I learned that the flowers were imperishable, and with such a wonderful discovery thrilling my spirit, I awoke.*[6]

Jastrow noted that Keller's dreams of seeing and hearing probably reflected conceptual interpretation, psychological apperception, or imaginative inference more than true sensation.[7] For adults with children who face severe physical or sensory challenges, it is important to understand that where there are severe limitations, dreams can arise to bring amazing experiences of moving into a realm of infinite possibilities.

Healing Dreams That Arise from Transformed Nightmares

Illness-related nightmares often disappear or transform as the anxiety and pain associated with the illness subsides. Nightmares at the onset of illness or at critical junctures in treatment sometimes take a positive turn and become healing dreams. For example, when 17-year-old Ron was first diagnosed with Hodgkin's lymphoma, he dreamed he was attacked by a menacing dark figure who wrestled him to the ground. A few months later, Ron dreamed the same attack, but this time he pinned the dark figure to the wall. Looking carefully into the face of his opponent, Ron saw the figure was crying and his face was Ron's own. Ron woke with a surprising feeling of compassion, and he vowed to befriend a part of himself who was still frightened and subject to tears.

Before her first radiation treatment, 10-year-old Beth had a nightmare about being alone and trapped inside a carnival haunted house. Before her second radiation treatment, Beth dreamed of walking up to the haunted house with her best friends. They talked and laughed as they bypassed the previously scary place, then headed for the Ferris wheel. Beth felt her second dream reflected her diminished fear of treatment.

Some nightmares transform on their own, but most nightmares transform as children are guided and companioned by caring adults who support them to engage in creative ways with the stresses, fears, anxieties, and pain of physical distress. Miguel was eight when he developed unexplainable gastrointestinal problems. Before going to the hospital for tests, he had a frightening dream.

> *I'm in a little boat. I fall into the big ocean. He's after me—the big shark with long, sharp teeth is eating me! Make him go away! I'm scared. Make him go away.*

Fortunately, Miguel's mother had learned some basic techniques for working with children's fears and was able to help her son calm down and get back to sleep. In the following days, using a combination of dreamplay tools, she helped him come to a new relationship with his fears.

Conscious Breathing

Paying attention to the breath is at the core of every practice for becoming calm, relaxed, centered, and focused. As breathing deepens and slows, it helps initiate the relaxation response which brings on conditions that are the exact opposite of the "fight or flight" response. Heart rate slows down, stress hormones subside, and endorphins that bring a sense of well-being increase. Activity moves from the rational to the intuitive part of the brain.[8] When a child is sick or in pain, she is usually quite willing to explore fun ways to breathe. When I was a special education teacher and consultant, I used two variations of slow, deep breathing that are helpful in calming an anxious child. The adult can demonstrate and then participate with the child. The goal is to practice together daily until the child is able to do the exercise on her own whenever she wants to calm herself.

- **Simply count the breaths:** Demonstrate breathing in deeply through the nose and releasing slowly through pursed lips while making a little sound. Breathe and count for as long as it takes the child to calm down. Help the child practice each day when he is not upset. Suggest that whenever he practices, to touch his heart or wrist. A physical gesture will serve as an anchor to reinforce relaxation whenever he practices the breathing exercise.

- **Belly breaths:** Diaphragmatic breathing helps children feel centered and calm. Educational psychologist Charlotte Reznick, in her book *The Power of Your Child's Imagination*,[9] calls this technique the *balloon breath*. "Let's take a few minutes to be aware of your breathing. Put your hands over your belly so you can notice your breath going there. That's right. Breathe slowly, about two to three inches just below your belly button, so your belly rises and falls as you breathe in and out. Good. Let's breathe in even slower, to the count of one ... two ... three. Now, breathe out just as slowly ... one ... two ... three." Reznick suggests practicing 1–3 minutes each session and repeating several times a day.

Progressive Relaxation

Deep, slow breathing is the first component of relaxation. Systematic relaxation of each part of the body is the second component. In the 1940s, Edmond Jacobson showed that when a person simply *imagined* moving or relaxing a specific muscle, its electrical energy changed.[10] Today, progressive relaxation is basic to many meditative approaches and children enjoy playful variations. When relaxed, a child can easily open the door to the imaginal realm to find resources for healing anxieties and transforming nightmares.

Using soft background music and speaking in a slow, soft voice, invite the child to focus on each part of her body from head to toes—first tensing the muscles and holding the tension for a moment, then releasing the tension and relaxing. This exercise helps children experience the difference between tension and relaxation. A full script can be found in Nancy Klein's book, *Healing Images for Children: Teaching Relaxation and Guided Imagery to Children Facing Cancer and Other Serious Illnesses.*[11]

Imaginal Progressive Relaxation

Many ill, injured, or handicapped children are unable to tense certain muscles but they still can benefit from a variation by simply imagining each part of the body relaxing. Starting with head or toes, invite the child to focus attention on each body part one by one and imagine each part becoming warm, soft, and relaxed. I do this exercise with adults at cancer centers. A full script can be found in my book on dreams and guided imagery.[12]

Gathering Healing Imagery

Imagery is much more than visualization. Imagery is apperception through any and all the senses plus the multiplicity of emotions and associations that arise in the presence of an image. When an image evokes a sense of safety, support, happiness, and hope we call it a healing image. Especially for children, healing images often speak louder than words.

When a child is physically distressed, remind him repeatedly of the things he loves and ask him to imagine and name them—animals: real, toy, and imaginal; beloved places, toys, books, activities, memories; his most-loved people; magical and spiritual beings. When a child is terrified, suggest she create one of her healing images through expressive art as a way to balance the scary emotions. Surround a sick child with her art pieces and photographs of her special people, things, and places. Let him keep within reach his precious possessions such as a shiny rock onto which he has projected magical qualities. Whether imagined or in concrete form, healing symbols carry energies for enhancing all the body's innate healing systems.[13]

There are many stories that illustrate the power of healing imagery. A good example is a story of a rag doll that influenced Emily's healing dreams for over 50 years. Another is a story of an ongoing photography project with teenagers who are hospitalized with chronic illness.

- **Compassionate healer with red hair:** When Emily was four; she broke her arm and was put in an adult ward because there were no nearby children's hospitals. Her arm was put in traction for six weeks. Emily's mother was not allowed to bring newborn baby sister to the hospital, and since there was no one else to watch the baby, Emily's only visitor was her father who came by twice a day to read to her. Emily remembers the pain, fear, and loneliness. She also holds vivid memories of the comfort brought by her Raggedy Ann doll. In her imagination, Emily and Raggedy Ann were in constant dialogue. The doll served as a compassionate friend and trusted guide throughout the hospital ordeal. When Emily was 15, she fractured her ankle and had her first dream of a beautiful red-haired woman with piercing black eyes who came to her as a loving, supportive companion. In her 20s, in times of illness, she had two more dreams of the beautiful red-haired healing helper. Emily is now almost 60 and has recorded six more similar dreams. At some point, she realized the connection between Raggedy Ann with her shaggy red hair and piercing black eyes and the beautiful healer who has come in dreams through the years.
- **Teen spirit:** Another example of the healing power of imagery is dramatically displayed in the photographs of hospitalized Atlanta teens with serious chronic illness. Once a month, for almost four years, a crew of volunteer professional photographers has helped seriously ill teens take pictures of one another to bring forth images of the people they want to be in spite of debilities and the pain of disease. The teens have also written about their feelings. One girl wrote, "I have Crohn's disease, but Crohn's most definitely doesn't have me." The photographs are not just pictures of smiling faces. A powerful

"portrait" is of a girl standing on one leg in colorful multicolored socks. The floor is on the diagonal, and she is visible only from the hips down. The result is "a vision of strength in an unstable world." In several public exhibits, people outside the hospital have been privileged to share the power and magic of the photography project, aptly called *Teen Spirit*.[14] As the project continues, more and more children are being helped to experience a transforming relationship to their serious illnesses.

Guided Imagery

Guided meditative journeys for healing have been practiced for centuries. In the present-day field of integrative medicine, guided imagery is used to enhance relaxation and sleep, explore and transform disturbing emotions and perceptions, prepare for procedures and surgery, reduce blood loss during surgery and the need for pain medicine afterwards. It is also used to reduce pain and the side effects of medical treatment such as nausea and fatigue. Among current experts in the field of guided imagery for integrative health care are Belleruth Naparstek and Martin Rossman, MD. Their books are classics in integrative wellness, and up-to-date research can be found on their websites.[15]

A guided imagery journey can induce a meditative state of consciousness and is a form of lucid waking dream in which "the dreamer" intentionally seeks support and an experience of new possibilities. With melodic, meditative music playing in the background, the "dreamer" is guided by an audio recording or an actual facilitating person to breathe and relax into a deep state of consciousness so that input from the associative, emotional, and intuitive parts of the brain can bring forth symbolic and metaphoric imagery that speaks in the same manner as a healing, sleeping dream.

Guided Imagery Journeys for Children

Almost always, children are enthusiastic subjects for imaginal journeying. If possible, use soft melodic background music to enhance the journey experience. Speak slowly with long pauses between each phrase. Mix and match the components that follow. Adjust vocabulary to the age and needs of the particular child. Add unique imagery you feel is helpful. Practice with the child daily.

- **Special healing place:** "Now imagine walking through a doorway and coming to a place that feels totally beautiful and safe. This is your own special place to come whenever you want to feel well. Open your eyes. Look all around and notice everything you see that helps you feel safe and comfortable. Open your ears. Listen. What sounds do you hear? Let the beautiful sounds soothe you. Are there good smells or tastes? Breathe them in. As you move around or sit or stand, reach out and touch what's near you. Feel the beauty and safety through your hands and breathe into your heart. Take deep breaths of warm energy for feeling happy and safe in this special place. When you're ready, take a deep, slow breath, wiggle your hands and feet; and come back noticing you feel centered and balanced."

- **Supportive allies:** "Now invite an ally to help you today. It might be someone you know, a hero from a book, movie or video, or helpful animal, wizard, or spiritual being who just pops in from your imagination. Keep your eyes closed, breathe deeply, relax, and let's just wait and see who shows up. Now invite your helper to be with you today. Feel safe and loved in the presence of your supporter. Breathe in the good feeling of love between you."

- **Imagery for reducing pain:** "Now that you're feeling relaxed and safe, go inside your body and locate where you're feeling pain. Imagine the place as a dark spot. Place your hand over the painful spot if you can, but even if you can't, every time you take a breath, simply imagine sending warm, healing light into any place in your body that needs love and care to feel better. Imagine the dark spot getting brighter and brighter as the pain becomes softer and softer and softer."

- **Imagery for surgery, chemotherapy, and other daunting medical challenges:** Scripts and commercial audio recordings for specific medical challenges are available from several sources.[16] You can also create your own script for a challenging situation. Start with deep breathing and relaxation; guide the child to a safe place and invite special supporters. Continue by inviting the child to imagine the challenge in a creative way that is helpful to getting well and feeling better. For example: Shauna imagines her chemotherapy infusion as water from a healing fountain. Her tumor shrinks in a magical spray. John imagines helpful little Martians zapping his tumor with rays from the radiation machine. Lorna imagines breathing in dragon power whenever she uses her asthma inhaler. Skipper lines up his daily pills and imagines them as tiny soldiers who storm and defeat his pesky virus.

- **Imagery for transforming nightmares:** A nightmare is a symbolic reflection of a child's underlying fear, anxiety, and pain, both physical and emotional. Nightmare images are uniquely personal and precise. Like the giant shark in Miguel's dream, vivid nightmare images can provide adults with a starting point for facilitating the child to deal creatively with underlying fear. If a nightmare has not brought imagery of a fearful challenge, then ask the child to go inside and imagine an image of whatever is frightening her. Encourage details. Once there is a clear, scary image, invite the child to get comfortable and to begin with breathing, relaxing, and going to a special place. Invite a supportive companion or companions. Then continue: "Now that your special animal/person/wizard/angel is here, ask him or her to guide you from the scary dream to a new dream where you feel good with yourself and with whatever is happening. Imagine you and your guide are watching the scary dream from behind a magic screen. You can see out, but no one can see in or get in. You are totally safe. Notice that the dream is changing. Some things are becoming different. New things are happening and you are feeling and acting in a new way. Watch carefully. Breathe in the good feelings for as long as you like. When you're ready to come back, promise yourself that when you're practicing your breathing and relaxing, you'll come back and reimagine this new dream. Promise yourself you'll enjoy the good feelings and new actions over and over again." (*Elements of a nightmare or symbolic images of a scary waking situation seldom change all at once. Repeat meditative dream reentry until the child feels a new relationship with the subject of his or her fear. When the dream transforms, rehearse the new dream often*).

Active Imagination/Imaginal Conversations

Younger children naturally talk to their toys and provide narration as toys talk to one another. Older children naturally express imaginal scenarios while they do imagery journeys, draw, and journal. There is deep wisdom for healing within every child and it is often expressed through dialogues with images of supportive allies as well as images of monsters. Children can dialogue with a personified image of a feeling such as pain, anger, fear, courage, hope, and love. They can also dialogue with a personified image of a body part such as a tumor, infected leg, paralyzed arm, or missing finger. Adults can encourage children of all ages to share their feelings through active imagination—to yell at Pain Monster, to cuddle Scaredy Cat, to tell Angry Dog to go chew on a bone. Adults can prompt with helpful questions: *What does Pain Monster need to feel better? Is there a color you can breathe in that will help him move away? What can your angel do for Scaredy Cat to give him more courage? If Angry Dog calms down, how might he be able to help you? What do you imagine Chemo Wizard might say about this? What might Wise Turtle do next?* The main job of adults is to encourage creative expression of all feelings and to affirm to the children that they are heard. Only when feelings are repressed do they contribute to illness.

All children naturally enact challenging situations through imagination and play. Several parents talked about their children rehearsing medical procedures with favorite toys. Bobby with juvenile diabetes gets to practice daily injections with a real syringe on a beloved stuffed animal. Trisha with third degree burns gets to "doctor" an injured doll with real dressings. All children are empowered by an opportunity to learn about, talk about, and play with equipment and devices needed for their medical care. "When they let me play with it, I can own it!" This statement was from Katie, age five, who was in and out of the hospital for the first six years of her life. Her grandmother praised the hospital personnel who never seemed rushed and who always took time to familiarize Katie and the family about details of her treatment.

Expressive Art

Many children's hospitals are integrating educational and stress reduction activities through creative use of art and music. Studies show beneficial physiological and emotional effects of integrating these activities with standard medical care. In the emerging field of Child Life Specialist, young professionals are being certified to facilitate both parents and their hospitalized children to tap into the therapeutic power of imaginative expression through art and play. The Child Life Council, certifying board for Child Life Specialists, reports reduced procedural and post-procedural pain as well as less emotional distress and fewer physiological complications with Child Life interventions.[17]

Art and writing go hand in hand with guided imagery and imaginal play. They provide tangible media for transforming emotional relationships with physical distress. The toddler who screamed, "Ants, ants!" during her fever-induced nightmare later was helped to make a picture of big black dots with a magic marker, then throw the paper in a trash can saying, "Ants all gone!"

After his Giant Shark nightmare and a guided dream reentry with his mother, Miguel made a series of drawings. The first depicted a tiny Miguel falling from a small boat with a huge shark poised to swallow him. The second drawing showed a big rope coming from the sky pulling Miguel from the water. The third showed a smiling giant Miguel standing on a boat while pointing down at a very small fish in the water. The nightmare and follow-up dream reentry plus art activities all contributed to reduced anxiety about his upcoming hospital visit.

Caring for a child facing illness, injury, or physical handicap can feel like an overwhelming task. Watching one's child suffer is very stressful, and the stress is compounded by knowing that how one's child will face a medical challenge is directly related to how the caregiving adult faces the challenge.[18] Fortunately, the time has arrived when practices such as dreamplay, art, and music are being integrated with standard medical care. These practices utilize the creative power of the imagination, and as a result, adults along with children are finding new, powerful resources that offer strength and hope for the healing journey.

Notes

1. Tallulah Lyons, *Dreams and Guided Imagery: Gifts for Transforming Illness and Crisis* (Bloomington, Indiana: Balboa Press, 2012), 119–143.

2. Carl G. Jung, *Collective Works of C. G. Jung, Volume 11: Psychology and Religion*, trans. Gerhard Adler and R.F.C. Hull (New Jersey: Princeton University Press, 2nd edition, 1970).

3. Billy Howard, introduction to *Angels and Monsters: A Child's Eye View of Cancer* by Lisa Murray (Atlanta: American Cancer Society, 2002), x.

4. Jeremy Taylor, *Wisdom of Your Dreams* (New York: Tarcher/Penguin, 2009), 265.

5. Richard Catlette Wilkerson, "Dreams of the Blind," *Electric Dreams* 2, 1, www.dreamgate.com/dream/ed-backissues/ed2-1.htm, accessed July 6, 2015.

6. Ibid.

7. Ibid.

8. Herbert Benson, *The Relaxation Response* (New York: Harper Torch, 1975).

9. Charlotte Reznick, *The Power of Your Child's Imagination: How to Transform Stress and Anxiety into Joy and Success* (New York: Penguin Group, 2009), 22.

10. Edmond Jacobson, *Progressive Relaxation* (Chicago: University of Chicago Press, 1938).

11. Nancy Klein, *Healing Images for Children: Facing Cancer and Other Serious Illness* (Watertown, WI: Inner Coaching, 2001), 42–44.

12. Lyons, *Dreams and Guided Imagery*, 33–34.

13. Martin L. Rossman, MD, *Fighting Cancer from Within* (New York: Henry Holt and Co., 2003), 19.

14. Catherine Fox, "Exhibit of Photographic Self-Portraits by Chronically Ill Kids, 'Teen Spirit' Will Raise Yours," November 6, 2012, review in *Atlanta Journal* newspaper: http://www.artsatl.com/2012/11/exhibit-photographic-self-portraits-chronically-ill-kids-teen-spirit-raise-yours/.

15. Belleruth Naparstek, *Staying Well with Guided Imagery* (New York: Time Warner Books, 1994). www.healthjourneys.com; Martin L. Rossman MD, *Fighting Cancer from Within* (New York: Henry Holt and Co., 2003). www.thehealingmind.org.

16. http://www.imageryforkids.com/; http://www.ipgbook.com/inner-coaching-publisher-INN.php; For teens and adults: http://www.healthjourneys.com/Storewww.healingpowerofdreams.com.

17. Child Life Council website: https://www.childlife.org/The%20Child%20Life%20Profession/, accessed July 6, 2015.

18. Child Life Council website: https://www.childlife.org/The%20Child%20Life%20Profession/, accessed July 6, 2015.

Bibliography

Benson, Herbert. *The Relaxation Response*. New York: Harper Torch, 1975.

Child Life Council website. Accessed July 6, 2015. https://www.childlife.org/The%20Child%20Life%20Profession/.

Dossey, Larry. *Healing Beyond the Body: Medicine and the Infinite Reach of the Mind.* Boston: Shambala Press, 2003.

Fox, Catherine. "Exhibit of Photographic Self-Portraits by Chronically Ill Kids, 'Teen Spirit' Will Raise Yours," November 6, 2012, review in *Atlanta Journal* newspaper. Accessed July 6, 2015. http://www.artsatl.com/2012/11/exhibit -photographic-self-portraits-chronically-ill-kids-teen-spirit-raise-yours/.

Garfield, Patricia. *The Healing Power of Dreams.* New York: Simon and Schuster, 1991.

Jacob, Edmonson. *Progressive Relaxation.* Chicago: University of Chicago Press, 1938.

Juvenile Diabetes website. Accessed July 6, 2015. http://www.t1everydaymagic .com/diabetes-art-projects-to-do-with-your-child/.

Jung, Carl G. *Collective Works of C. G. Jung, Volume 11: Psychology and Religion.* Translated by Gerhard Adler and R.F.C. Hull. New Jersey: Princeton University Press, 2nd edition, 1970.

Klein, Nancy. *Healing Images for Children: Facing Cancer and Other Serious Illness.* Watertown, WI: Inner Coaching, 2001.

Lasley, Justina. *Wake Up to Your Dreams.* Double Spiral Publishing, 2015.

Lyons, Tallulah. *Dreams and Guided Imagery: Gifts for Transforming Illness and Crisis.* Bloomington, IN: Balboa Press, 2012.

Murray, Lisa, and Billy Howard. *Angels and Monsters: A Child's Eye View of Cancer.* Atlanta, GA: American Cancer Society, 2002.

Naparstek, Belleruth. *Staying Well with Guided Imagery.* New York: Time Warner Books, 1994.

Newman, Zoe. *Lucid Waking: Using Dreamwork Principles to Transform Your Everyday Life.* Berkeley, CA: White Egret Press, 2010.

Norment, Rachel, *Guided by Dreams: Breast Cancer, Dreams, and Transformation.* Richmond: Brandylane Publishers, 2006.

Reznick, Charlotte. *The Power of Your Child's Imagination: How to Transform Stress and Anxiety into Joy and Success.* New York: Penguin Group, 2009.

Rossman, Martin. *Fighting Cancer from Within.* New York: Henry Holt and Co., 2003.

Siegel, Alan and Kelly Bulkeley. *Dreamcatching: Every Parent's Guide to Exploring and Understanding Children's Dreams and Nightmares.* New York: Three Rivers Press, 1998.

Shapiro, Lawrence E. and Robin K. Sprague. *The Relaxation and Stress Reduction Workbook for Kids.* Oakland, CA: Instant Help Books, 2009.

Taylor, Jeremy. *The Wisdom of Your Dreams: Using Dreams to Tap into Your Unconscious and Transform Your Life.* New York: Tarcher/Penguin, 2009.

Wilkerson, Richard Catlette. "Dreams of the Blind." *Electric Dreams* 2(1). Accessed July 6, 2015. http://www.dreamgate.com/dream/articles_rcw/ed2-1bli.htm.

PART TWO
Inner and Outer Worlds

Dragons, Angels, and Rites of Passage: The Universal Language of Children's Dreams

Angel Morgan

[I] was in a very big and special chair.... Nine people, who seemed more like angels, came ... through a mist of glittering light. Each brought ... a special gift.
Lynn, age 4[1]

Dreaming is a universal language that unites all people regardless of cultural, historical, and social differences. In the world of dreams, dragons can represent important lessons that children, teens, and adults can learn from their dreams: to face fears, integrate animal instincts, tame antisocial behavior, and feel empowered to soar to great heights. Angels appear in many forms in young people's dreams, often to help integrate spiritual guidance, parental guidance, and teacher guidance. Rites of passage dreams of universal importance will be outlined here so that parents, caregivers, and other professionals working with youth, can better understand how these experiences make young people feel and how to recognize and honor them when they happen. Adults can help improve children's lives by consciously recognizing developmental dream opportunities and guiding children to act upon them.

Within this chapter, the theories of Swiss developmental psychologist Jean Piaget[2] and Austrian philosopher Rudolf Steiner,[3] founder of Waldorf

Education, will be used as frames of reference for the practical dream work and dreamplay techniques I share. In over two decades as a parent, dream worker, Waldorf teacher, and research psychologist specializing in dreams and creativity, I developed The Dreambridge Dream-Arts Curriculum.[4] Using the child development theories of Piaget and Steiner, I will outline some age-appropriate activities from this curriculum.

Negative language about dreams in Western culture has perpetuated negative associations. Books and movies speak about having "bad dreams" or tell child characters that "it was just a dream," or "only a dream." When something bad happens, we exclaim: "What a nightmare!" These negative references to dreams have become so ingrained that people may not even realize they are belittling one of our primary states of consciousness. When we recognize we have been culturally belittling dreams, we can also decide that we have the power to change those habits. All dreams are actually good if we understand that they speak in a dream language that can be learned, and that they come in the service of healing and wholeness.[5]

In the service of children of all ages, let us now go fearlessly toward the heart of the dream dragon.

Dreaming with Young Children around the World

Dreams mirror waking life development,[6] and also influence waking life development,[7] so making dream sharing fun and natural for children is important. Although they often share dreams as soon as they can speak in their mother tongue, young children are not always able to articulate what they have been dreaming. That does not mean that their dream experiences are any less profound or important. The ability to describe dreams usually evolves at the same intensity and pace in which children develop language capacities while they are awake.[8]

However, because development is not purely linear, we may also lose certain capacities we had as children as we grow older. Every night children sleep and dream, and dream opportunities offer them potential gifts. With every developmental gift that children unwrap on their path toward adulthood, they also leave behind some of childhood's magic with the wrapping paper.

Ordinary dreams speak in a universal language of puzzles. Some dream puzzles can take many years for dreamers to solve. Most dream sentences are formed with symbols, metaphors, and puns. For example, a mother set the intention to cut all unhealthy cords between herself and her daughter that were burdening their relationship. Early the next morning, the child awoke crying and reported this dream:

I'm in the water and Mom is in the back of the boat. She has an old rope that she is pulling away from me. I'm reaching for it, but I can't get it. There's a ring [life buoy] that I'm holding onto.

Julie, age 5[9]

It can take a while for each dreamer to learn this language fluently, especially since there are such a wide variety of translations for dreamers to choose from. Dreamers of any age determine the final translations. Within the universal dream language, one's culture and personal mythology[10] make a difference when decoding it.

Complexity may be experienced in dreams at a very young age, when children are not yet able to articulate what they experienced. For example, when Carl Jung was between three and four years old, he had a big dream:

It was a magnificent throne, a real king's throne in a fairy tale. Something was standing on it which I thought at first was a tree trunk twelve to fifteen feet high and about one and a half to two feet thick. It was a huge thing, reaching almost to the ceiling. But it was of a curious composition: it was made of skin and naked flesh, and on top there was something like a rounded head with no face and no hair. On the very top of the head was a single eye, gazing motionlessly upward.... The thing did not move, yet I had the feeling that it might at any moment crawl off the throne like a worm and creep toward me. I was paralyzed with terror.[11]

It was not until Jung was an adult that he felt he understood this dream's meaning in his life. He reflected, "This dream haunted me for years. Only much later did I realize that what I had seen was a phallus, and it was decades before I understood that it was a ritual phallus."[12] That he could not describe this dream experience in such vivid detail until he was an adult is important. It reminds us that sometimes little children dream big, and they cannot always comfortably report much of what they experience during sleep.

Young children generally think through doing, and learn through imitation,[13] so what parents and educators say and do is important modeling for children under seven. They usually feel most comfortable sharing their dreams with a close relative, due to their need for safety, comfort, and trust during this powerfully open and vulnerable stage of life. When addressing children and their inner worlds, it is important to respect their journey. The opportunity to guide children and their dream development is a great honor.

Here are two questions that are useful for adults to ask themselves before beginning dreamplay with children:

- Are my words and actions worthy of a young child's imitation?[14]
- Do I model dream sharing with children in a positive and fun way?

Some societies, such as the Senoi Temiar of Malaysia,[15] the Guarani of Brazil,[16] the Mapuche of Chile,[17] Tibetan monks, Australian Aborigines, and many other indigenous cultures such as Native American tribes have practiced sharing, discussing dreams with children, and offering culturally specific guidance.[18] In the film, *A Dreamer and the Dream Tribe*, Awin Pedik, a member of the Senoi Temiar tribe says,

> If a dream comes every night, then we will discuss the matter every day. And then as a result when these children are grown up, whatever they dream they can interpret by themselves. Sometimes they go to the shaman and seek his advice, because sometimes the dreams of small children may send an important message to the community.[19]

American parapsychologist Stanley Krippner's research tells us that in Guarani culture, "a child can have a dream that indicates a new direction for a community"[20] and that in Mapuche culture, "Most Mapuche dream interpretation is conducted within the family each morning and before important events."[21]

In the documentary film, *The Power of Dreams, Part III: Sacred Sleep*,[22] Australian aboriginal children are shown dancing in a natural setting, learning through storytelling that the world was created in "The Dreamtime" long ago through story, dance, and song. Later in the same film, some 10-year-old boys living in a Tibetan monastery tell their dreams to the abbot because their dreams inform him what teaching they are prepared to comprehend. No matter what society you live in, you can help normalize dream sharing and make it a positive, empowering experience for children.

A common adult reaction to children's dream sharing, especially when the dream seems "bad" by cultural standards, is to say, "It wasn't real. It was just a dream." According to Piaget's Preoperational Stage (see Table 5.1), for children ages two to seven who are not yet able to conceptualize abstractly and need concrete physical situations,[23] dreams and nightmares are very real. The magical thinking phase of the young child, in which a three-year-old believes that it rains, "so the flowers can grow"[24] is natural and healthy. It helps young children develop the confidence they need to be creative later in life.[25]

The Dream-Arts Curriculum in Table 5.1 emphasizes adults in young children's lives learning about dreams and nightmares, modeling positive dream sharing, and guiding physical dream arts activities such as drawing or painting a dream, and dream puppet shows.

Table 5.1 Theories of Piaget and Steiner in Correspondence to Morgan's Dream-Arts Curriculum

Piaget's Stages	Steiner's Rhythms	Morgan's Curriculum
Ages 2–7	Ages 0–7	Ages 0–7
Preoperational Stage: Child not yet able to conceptualize abstractly and needs concrete physical situations	The young child thinks through doing, and learns through imitation.	Parent Dream Education: Pro-empowerment, anti-fear. Dream Art Dream Puppet Theater

Approaching dreams by not approaching them is not the best choice. Although they may change in form, nightmares do not disappear until they are faced. Facing nightmares, and transforming fear into empowerment, is a skill that can be learned and developed over time.

If a child does not learn to face her dragons in dreams, when she goes to school it can feel extremely difficult for her to confidently call upon the self-esteem she needs to face a bully, or grow out of a tendency to bully others. It does not comfort children to say dreams are not real, or that they are insignificant (just a dream). That teaches them to be more afraid because they know and feel that they experienced something more powerful and real than what they are being told. When young children share scary dreams, it is beneficial to remind them that they are not alone, and that they will grow stronger.

When I was a young child, my father was my first dream guide. I continued this tradition when raising my own (now adult) children. Teaching children about dreams as they grow and develop not only empowers them, it also strengthens and deepens your relationship with them. When my son was a high school freshman, I asked him if he remembered my dream guidance when he first experienced nightmares. In the "Luke on Dreambridge" YouTube video, he explains:

> At first it was a little confusing and I almost didn't get it. But you know, after the first couple of nightmares, they almost didn't even seem like nightmares! And I could almost even not have to come to your room. I could just sort of try to figure it out myself and go back to bed.[26]

Lucid Dreaming: The Bridge between Dreams and Waking Life

When I was four and my father taught me about dreams, he primarily relied on Kilton Stewart's[27] model for dream education based on what

Stewart learned from the Senoi Temiar tribe in the 1930s. With the guidance of dream allies, I began to develop my inner capacities just as Stewart claimed the Senoi children did. By the time I was 19 and studying with Stewart's widow, Clara, I was a very lucid dreamer. However, when I was just four I awoke from a nightmare and called for my dad. After reassuring me, he said,

> "The next time you have a nightmare, look for a Friendly Giant to protect you. When you need him, just whistle. You know how to whistle, right?"

When I went back to sleep, the nightmare returned. I woke up, and started whistling. I whistled for a few minutes before storming into my dad's room, announcing,

"I whistled and whistled, and you never came!"

I had imagined my dad was the giant, as he was very tall compared to me, and the friendliest giant I knew. After walking me back to bed, he explained to me that I could call upon him or any other ally when I was still in a dream, or reentering a dream. He taught me that anything I needed to help me in my dream adventures, I could imagine. Eventually, I could do things myself that I had needed dream allies to help me with before. Most importantly, my fear went away without trying to make the dreams go away.

Dream allies can be parental figures, teachers, siblings, pets, or best friends. They can be favorite fictional characters such as superheroes, friendly wizards and witches, or other fantasy beings such as fairies, elves, dwarves, giants, sprites, gnomes, and angels. Favorite stuffed animals and dolls can make great dream allies, too.

Young children under the age of seven often dream about animals. They also dream a lot about being chased. Often, it is an animal in some form that is doing the chasing. Dreams of being chased give children opportunities to face their own animal instincts, and tame antisocial behavior in waking life.[28] However, when this rite of passage is not recognized and guided at the outset, chasing dreams can continue for years. An older boy in India had this dream:

> *I am walking and suddenly a dog starts chasing me. I am terrified if the dog bites me I will have 14 injections. I start crying.*
>
> Anshu, age 11[29]

There are many variables that come along with living a social life, and stress from waking life finds expression in children's nightmares. It helps to explain that being "number one in the dream" means all of your needs and wishes can be fulfilled in dreams.

When children feel that their needs are met in dreams, they feel more content in waking life from the inside out. In case you are wondering if that would teach children to be selfish or tyrannical, the opposite is actually true. Imagine feeling you are number one in your own dreams. When we are able to resolve conflict and experience inner peace in dreams, we can feel empowered to become more selfless, considerate, and generous to others in waking life. Meanwhile, suffering in dreams can make us feel less available socially in waking life because our deepest, subconscious needs have not been met.

As soon as children realize within the dream, that they are dreaming, they cross a threshold into what is called *lucid dreaming*, and doors to many creative possibilities open up. For example, falling dreams can turn into flying dreams.[30]

> *I am flying like a bird while the moon is shining and some birds are also awakened and flying with me.*
>
> Amit, age 8[31]

It helps to tell children about flying in dreams as a strategy for escaping fearful situations, especially before they find the courage to face what is chasing them in the dream. It is also helpful to tell children:

- Whatever chases you is a part of you (your dreaming mind).
- Whatever animal or monster, it probably has a gift for you when you feel ready to find out what it is.

> *The earliest dream I remember was about a yellow dragon that could breathe fire out of its tail, nose, mouth and left foot.*
>
> Cathy, age 8[32]

Children can learn how to transform dream dragons into friends and allies. For example, a British-German toddler reported a recurring nightmare to her mother in this simple language:

> *Dragon—sharp teeth!*
>
> Yazzie, age 2.5

Her mother, lucid dream researcher and coeditor of this book, Clare Johnson, taught her an empowering mantra, bought her a stuffed dragon to sleep with, and told her if she called for help in a scary dream then help would arrive. She encouraged her to befriend her dream dragons. When she was almost three, Yazzie reported: "Last night there was a laser-eyed dragon!" with empowerment instead of fear.[33]

This rite of passage may begin earlier or later, depending on the child. Younger children may need to call upon their allies to help them in lucid dreams for some time before feeling empowered enough by dream guidance to face their fears.

Since the change from milk teeth to adult teeth marks a rite of passage for increased learning capacities in the life of a child,[34] dreams about losing teeth (at any age) could symbolize preparing to learn something new. They could also represent feeling stressed, or needing to see a dentist. As universal as its stages may be, there are multiple ways to read specific "words" or "sentences" in the language of dreams.

From ages 7 to 11, children enter a stage Piaget called Concrete Operations[35] (see Table 5.2). During this stage, as physical experience accumulates, children start to conceptualize, creating logical structures that explain their physical experiences. However true, this does not describe the whole experience of the child. Steiner's perspective was that from age 7 to 14, children think in pictures, and learn through their feelings.[36]

The Dream-Arts Curriculum in Table 5.2 helps growing children creatively connect their inner dream world to the physical world. It helps them reflect on, share, and discuss what they learn about the bridge between dreams and waking life.

Betty Staley, a Waldorf educator and teacher training director at the Rudolf Steiner College, described in *Between Form and Freedom*[37] that with children these ages:

Table 5.2 Theories of Piaget and Steiner in Correspondence to Morgan's Dream-Arts Curriculum

Piaget's Stages	Steiner's Rhythms	Morgan's Curriculum
Ages 7–11	Ages 7–14	Ages 7–10
Concrete Operations: As physical experience accumulates, the child starts to conceptualize, creating logical structures that explain his or her physical experiences.	The child thinks in pictures and learns through the feelings.	Listen to and Re-tell: Multi-cultural dream stories. Drawing, painting, collage from dream stories. Older children write stories, poems, and plays from dream stories. Dream Journaling.

> The feeling life is developed in private, in a world of dreams, hopes, and fantasies. As their inner worlds develop depth, children begin to have secrets. The two worlds—the inner private and the outer public—interact, causing tension as children slowly learn to feel comfortable in both worlds. ... As children experience their new feelings, they show an increased interest in adventure stories. They relish the swing of emotions that they experience while listening to or reading a story filled with terror and suspense.[38]

As children develop new capacities in waking life, they become more capable to actively participate in lucid dream adventures. Simply suggesting a possibility can be enough for them to experience it that same night.

For example, lucid dream researcher Ed Kellogg wrote a challenge[39] for children to become lucid in a dream, and try to cast one of the spells from the *Harry Potter* series to see what happens. Both my children tried it. The next morning, my son told me that he had gotten as far as holding a wand, but before he could cast a spell, he was distracted by other events in his dream. At the time, he was 10. My daughter, who was 13, walked down the stairs and announced, "I did it! In my dream, I entered a dark room, and made my wand light up the area by saying, '*Lumos!*' "

Within this age range, there is enormous potential to develop one's relationship with dreams, which are vivid in pictures, and rich in feelings. Applications of new, powerful dream lessons from dream guides can begin now.

Becoming a Dreamtime Warrior

The film *How to Train Your Dragon*[40] is an excellent analogy for a child's dream journey to face fears, integrate animal instincts, tame antisocial behavior, and feel empowered to soar to great heights. The main character starts out weak and fearful (the young child), then learns to face his fears by connecting with the dragon (his own animal instincts) that was once perceived as a powerful threat to his community (taming antisocial behavior). He helps the dragon, names it, and learns to ride it in a way that is quite natural for lucid dreamers (dreamtime warrior). He shows everyone else how to train dragons rather than kill them (transforming dragons). He gains an entirely new relationship to dragons, and no longer fears them. From this achievement, he becomes a confident, strong, loved hero in his community (lucid dreams affect waking life, too).

Over two decades ago, a similar story was told to me by Clara, the widow of Kilton Stewart. Stewart had told her about the lucid dreaming lessons Senoi Temiar children received from their parents as Dream Guides in the 1930s. However, for the Senoi Temiars, it was not dragons that were feared but tigers living in the jungle. When children eventually learned how to transform, befriend, and ride upon a tiger's back in their dreams it was a sign of their development both in lucid dreams and in waking life. What children have to work with from their cultures in waking life influences the universal pattern of what is possible when these opportunities appear. The idea is to help them recognize the opportunity, and engage in creative, imaginative dreamplay.

For example, I tell a Senoi-inspired story to children about Taio-m the dream warrior, and his tiger, Sido-t. Children love to hear various cultural dream stories, rich in imagery and feeling, based on views of the dreamtime that have been passed down from our ancestors by oral and written traditions. When you light up while telling a story that incorporates dream wisdom with a dash of adventure, your audience of children will, too.

A day or two after hearing a dream story is a great time for the children to draw, paint, or collage what they took in and imagined from the stories. This allows a healthy, natural weaving between inner and outer experience, while providing a primary education about dreams. Children closer to nine and ten years old become more capable of rewriting or telling the story in their own words, writing a poem, song, or play about the dream story, and extending dream stories in empowering ways.

These activities prepare them to work with and share their own dreams artistically, when they feel ready to do so. It is helpful by this age to encourage children to start writing in their own dream journal.

To help children of any age become dreamtime warriors, when they report nightmares, first acknowledge that something just happened to them that felt scary. Then reassure them:

- You are brave and you have dream allies.
- Your favorite superheroes will help you in your dreams if "the bad guys" return.
- You are safe in your dreams, and do not need to feel afraid.
- You are the dreamer, and number one in the dream.
- Everyone in your dream should be helpful and friendly to you.

Dreamtime warriors can:

- Practice facing opposing forces with courage.
- Find a good place to land after flying in dreams, and feel bare feet touch the earth (very grounding in waking life).
- Create a magic backpack that holds anything they need by simply imagining it (like Mary Poppins's carpetbag).
- Make things happen, appear, and change in dreams, simply by thinking about it.
- Use a magic wand to be creative, or a lightsaber to protect themselves and others on their dream adventures.

- Practice spells from famous characters such as *Harry Potter*, *Merlin*, and *Morgan Le Fay*.

The Special Needs of Teen Dreamers

Piaget called the stage from ages 11 to 15 Formal Operations (see Table 5.3), indicating that the child's cognitive structures are now like those of an adult and include conceptual reasoning.[41] However, cognitive structures are not the whole experience of a young person. Years of experience and maturity add to the gradual differentiations between a preteen, a teen, and an adult. Steiner pointed out that just as physical reproductive capacities mature, the preteen of 11 to 13 becomes more capable of expanding her intellectual capacities.[42]

With the onset of puberty, young people enter into what Steiner called a phase of negation. They suddenly experience the world differently, and have changing needs. For those in the negation phase, pushing away from the outer world often coincides with a pulling in (retreating) toward the dream world. Young teens usually feel ready and willing to share their dreams with other peers they feel safe with, and enjoy exploring their dream content creatively.

The Dream-Arts Curriculum in Table 5.3 guides teens to create more sophisticated dream bridges and a healthy social life as they travel along the path to adulthood.

In order to build upon lucid dreaming skills and become more familiar with the bridge between waking and dreaming experience, young teens

Table 5.3   Theories of Piaget and Steiner in Correspondence to Morgan's Dream-Arts Curriculum

Piaget's Stages	Steiner's Rhythms	Morgan's Curriculum
Ages 11–15	Onset of Puberty	Ages 11–13
Formal Operations: The child's cognitive structures are like those of an adult and include conceptual reasoning.	Negation Phase: Opposing, refuting, criticizing the world.	Active Re-dreaming, Lucid Dreaming, Dream Art, Dream Writing/ Poetry, Improvisational Dream Theater, Dream Journal
	Ages 16–17	Ages 14–17
	Affirmation Phase: Adolescents try to find their way into the life of the outer world.	Dream Circle Protocols, Tools for Transforming Nightmares, Creative Writing from Dreams or Nightmares.

can practice actively re-dreaming in daydreams. Because of more complex thinking, it can become habitual for teens to ask dream figures who they are, what they want, and see what answers they receive.

Dream arts continue to offer valuable modes of expression that can expand at this time. Dream poetry starts to take a different tone that is reflected in part by the maturing dream poet, sometimes revealing a much older soul. Teens that are new to exploring their dreams (as well as adults) can also reveal slightly younger seeming dreams due to rites of passage that were previously ignored. As Stewart wrote, "In the West the thinking we do while asleep usually remains on a muddled, childish, or psychotic level because we do not respond to dreams as socially important and include dreaming in the educative process."[43] Dream arts hold great value for teens whether they received dream guidance as a child, or are just getting started now.

A new way to honor the dream and the dreamer at this time is with Improvisational Dream Theater. Acting is a wonderful outlet for preteens and teens because their feeling life after puberty can be so intense. Dreams, rich in feeling and emotional expression, are now well expressed theatrically. Acting dreams out, and then again as a re-dream can be very empowering and fun at this stage. As the group's dream guide, explain that the dreamer gets to be the director, and you are there to assist them.

In a class I taught with a group of young teens, a 13-year-old I will call Ruby first told us her dream:

> *I'm in a green room with a loveseat and coffee table. I'm being chased around the furniture by a dragon and a little trollish looking person. We keep running in circles around and around. I'm screaming for help.*

I asked her to cast the others in the class to play her dream characters. Ruby cast herself as herself, a boy as the loveseat, another boy as the dragon, and a girl as the troll. She cast me to play the role of the coffee table. Then she directed us to act out the dream.

After we acted it out, I asked Ruby how she felt.

"Scared. Helpless. Silly."
"What would happen if you turned around and faced them?"
"I don't know. They might eat me!"
"Do you want me to help you?"
"You're a coffee table!"
"Yes, but in dreams, coffee tables can help you. Do you want me to?"
"Yes!"

We turned to face the dragon and troll, and they turned and started running the other way. Following Ruby's lead, we started running after them. The dragon and troll yelled out:

"Help! Don't get us!"
Ruby yelled:
"Stop! We're not going to hurt you!"

We all laughed and fell to the floor. I advised Ruby to offer her hand in friendship, and to tell her new friends they are now her allies.

Dreams about love interests and sex start happening more for young people after crossing the threshold of puberty. They also dream a lot about their crushes. Sometimes, romantic or sexual dreams happen because they feel attracted to their crushes physically in waking life. Other times, their crushes have talents and qualities that they identify with, respect, or admire, and would like to integrate into their own personalities. Sometimes, it is both. When dreams like these are shared, it helps to ask the teen, "What is it about that friend, movie star, or musician that you like?" and, "How would you like to be more like that?" It is very positive for teens to dream about their crushes, because it helps them form their own identities, get in touch with their values, and learn what kind of people they want to be as they grow up into a much larger world.

Classic wet dreams are completely natural, normal, and healthy. If a young person tells you he had this experience, usually it is because he feels afraid and in need of some reassurance. The best way to handle a situation like this is to remain calm and unsurprised by it. Once you know what he is asking about, it is best not to ask questions beyond what he wants to tell you. You can say something simple and reassuring such as, "Dreams like that are completely natural, normal, and healthy." Remaining as unfazed as possible by the topic of sex can be difficult for many adults.

Around the age of 16, teens enter what Steiner called the phase of affirmation. Staley wrote, "At this point, adolescents begin to search . . . for a picture of the world with which they can be comfortable."[44] During this phase, dream work and dreamplay should be focused to help teenagers strengthen the relationship between their (inner) dream worlds and (outer) waking-life worlds.

Through the social act of participating in a dream circle, teens learn to develop a common dream vocabulary while cultivating compassion and open-mindedness to the experience of others. They can bridge their dreams creatively into the social realm by sharing individual experiences and collaborating.

After practicing lucid dreaming, a teen can feel prepared to instinctively face opposing forces in his or her dreams. A classic film portrayal of lucidity after previously feeling under attack is in *The Matrix*[45] when Neo becomes fearless, faces the enemy that is chasing him and stops bullets with his mind. Another is in Tim Burton's version of *Alice in Wonderland*[46] when Alice faces the Jabberwocky because she no longer fears it and realizes she is the one (the dreamer).

It is normal for teenagers to experience nightmares about death, because they are growing fast toward adulthood, and going through many changes. Dreams that feel negative can often symbolize this growth and change—and on the contrary, be very positive. Apocalyptic nightmares can symbolize that a teen dreamer's entire world is dramatically changing in waking life.

> *I'm on an island. Fighter planes are flying overhead. Bombs are dropping from inside the planes, exploding everywhere.*
>
> Akasha, 16[47]

In the heat of a nightmare, it can be difficult to see what it is all about, but when teens take time with their nightmare images to gain clarity, it helps them grow emotionally. It is helpful for dream guides to discuss such death and destruction dreams with teens, and suggest they imagine the transformation completing with something new coming to life in its place—a rebirthing of dream energy.

A 16-year-old girl told me, "I've had a lot of dreams that I die? And like, I'm actually dying ... or like, it's my funeral or something." After I explained to her that death scenarios in ordinary dreams are often a metaphor for changes happening in waking life, she laughed in relief. Too many teenagers fear ordinary dreams about death because they have not been educated about the language of dreams.

Dream guides can explain to teens that *ordinary* dreams speak in puzzles using symbols, metaphors, and puns. Dream guides need to listen deeply in case a dream turns out to be what dream researchers call *extraordinary* dreams in addition to lucid ones, such as: dreams within dreams, out-of-body, telepathic, precognitive, clairvoyant, collective, past life, initiation, spiritual, or visitation dreams.[48] It is easier for people who have experienced extraordinary dreams to detect them in others (or believe in them). It is best to give children and teens of all ages the benefit of the doubt, and listen to their concerns with an open mind.

Expressing dream and nightmare content in creative writing, drama, and other dream arts can meet deep emotional needs for teens. Dreams can help teens by informing visual artwork, intentions of characters in plays, musical compositions, and film scripts. Adolescence is not known for being easy—its ups and downs can feel both thrilling and terrifying, like a roller coaster. Teens look forward to expanding their knowledge and experiences. Dream arts help them to master their inner roller coaster, and find creative expression at the same time.

For teenagers new to lucid dreaming, here is an imaginative exercise to build lucid *muscles* so they can feel prepared for more advanced, creative, and playful lucid dreaming adventures. Tell them:

> As you prepare to go to sleep tonight, imagine that you are standing at the bottom of a cliff in a warm, beautiful landscape. Look around and notice all of the details. Take a moment to feel the earth under your bare feet. Imagine levitating up to the top of the cliff and landing there. Then turn around to face the edge and imagine jumping off the cliff and slowly, gently, landing down at the bottom where you began. Once again, feel the earth beneath your feet.

They can repeat this exercise again and again until they fall asleep. The lucid workout helps teenagers experience how in lucid dreams the laws of physics do not apply the same ways they do in waking life. It helps them understand the important role the mind plays with experiences in dreams. In lucid dreams we can consciously choose to levitate, fly, and then land gently on the earth without a scratch. In waking life this can translate as: going up into the intellect, exploring inner space, and taking care to feel grounded again after all that adventure.

What will be the wider social impact of adults working thoughtfully with children's dreams? When my son was 14, I asked him a similar question. He said:

> A lot of kids have nightmares, and parents will just be like, "You had a bad dream, suck it up—go back to bed." . . . they just really don't know how to help them. I feel like if parents had [dream education] . . . it would really just help them explain to their child what's going on in the dream. And help them understand that a nightmare isn't always a bad thing. . . . Maybe there'd be a lot less bullying . . . people would be a lot kinder . . . probably just be a better world.[49]

It is my hope that many adult "angels" or dream guides working with children and teens will learn from the materials presented here. With more informed dream guides, more children and teens will learn to speak the empowering, universal language of dreams—and help us cocreate a better world.

Notes

1. Tobin Hart, *The Secret Spiritual World of Children* (Novato, CA: New World Library, 2003), 187.

2. Jean Piaget, *The Psychology of the Child* (New York: Basic, 2000).

3. Rudolf Steiner, *The Kingdom of Childhood* (New York: Anthroposophic Press, 1995).

4. "Dreambridge Workshops & Courses," http://thedreambridge.com/workshops.htm, accessed March 25, 2015.

5. Jeremy Taylor, *Where People Fly and Water Runs Uphill* (New York: Warner, 1992).

6. David Foulkes, *Children's Dreaming and the Development of Consciousness* (Cambridge, MA: Harvard University Press, 1999).

7. Kilton Stewart, "Mental Hygiene and World Peace," in *Mental Hygiene* 38, 1954: 387–403.

8. Foulkes, *Children's Dreaming.*

9. Hart, *The Secret Spiritual World*, 250.

10. David Feinstein and Stanley Krippner, *The Mythic Path*, 3rd ed. (Santa Rosa, CA: Elite, 2006).

11. Carl G. Jung, *Memories, Dreams, Reflections*, ed. Aniela Jaffé, trans. Richard and Clara Winston (New York: Vintage, 1989), 11–12.

12. Ibid., 17.

13. Steiner, *The Kingdom of Childhood*, 17–20.

14. Ibid., 19.

15. Arto Halonen, *A Dreamer and the Dream Tribe* (New York: Mystic Fire Video, 1998), VHS.

16. Stanley Krippner, "Anyone Who Dreams Partakes in Shamanism," *Journal of Shamanic Practice* 2(2), 2009: 33–40.

17. Barbara Tedlock, "Dreams" in *Encyclopedia of Religion*, 2nd ed., vol. 4, ed. L. Jones (Detroit, MI: Macmillan Reference USA, 2005), 2482–2491.

18. Angel Morgan, "Dream Sharing as a Healing Method: Tropical Roots and Contemporary Community Potential," *Journal of Tropical Psychology* 4(12), 2014: 1–16.

19. Halonen, *Dreamer and the Dream Tribe.*

20. Stanley Krippner, Fariba Bogzaran, and André Percia de Carvalho, *Extraordinary Dreams and How to Work with Them* (New York: SUNY Press, 2002), 34.

21. Ibid., 37.

22. The Discovery Channel, *The Power of Dreams, Part III: Sacred Sleep* (Silver Spring, MD: Discovery Communications, 1994), VHS.

23. Piaget, *Psychology of the Child.*

24. Stanley Krippner and Allan Combs, "Structures of Consciousness and Creativity: Opening the Doors of Perception," in *Everyday Creativity*, ed. Ruth Richards (Washington, DC: APA, 2007), 135.

25. Ibid., 137.

26. "Luke on Dreambridge," YouTube video, 4:37, posted by "TheDREAM-BRIDGE," https://www.youtube.com/watch?v=kGlf2I3VYlE, accessed June 23, 2013.

27. Kilton Stewart, "Dream Theory in Malaya," in *Altered States of Consciousness*, ed. Charles T. Tart (New York: Doubleday, 1969), 161–170.

28. Ibid.

29. Patricia Garfield, *Your Child's Dreams* (New York: Ballantine Books, 1984), 112.

30. Stewart, "Dream Theory in Malaya," 164–165.

31. Garfield, *Your Child's Dreams*, 263.

32. Brenda Mallon, *Dream Time with Children* (London: Jessica Kingsley, 2002), 28.

33. Private correspondence, September 2015.

34. Steiner, *Kingdom of Childhood*, 7–14.

35. Piaget, *Psychology of the Child*.

36. Rudolf Steiner, *Education of the Child in the Light of Anthroposophy* (London: Rudolf Steiner Press, 1965).

37. Betty Staley, *Between Form and Freedom* (Stroud, UK: Hawthorn Press, 1988).

38. Ibid., 5.

39. Ed Kellogg, "Harry Potter and the Lucid Dream Exchange Challenge: Trying out Spells from the Hogwarts Universe," *The Lucid Dream Exchange* 24–26, no. 36, September, 2005: http://www.dreaminglucid.com/using-magic-like-harry-potter/.

40. *How to Train Your Dragon*, directed by Dean De Blois and Chris Sanders (2010; North Hollywood: Dreamworks Animated, 2014), DVD/Blu-ray.

41. Piaget, *Psychology of the Child*.

42. Rudolf Steiner, *Education for Adolescents* (Barrington, MA: Anthroposophic Press, 1996).

43. Stewart, "Dream Theory in Malaya," 170.

44. Staley, *Between Form and Freedom*, 12.

45. *The Matrix*, directed by Andy Wachowski and Lana Wachowsky (1999; Burbank: Warner Bros., 1999), DVD.

46. *Alice in Wonderland*, directed by Tim Burton (2010; Burbank: Walt Disney Pictures, 2010), DVD.

47. My daughter, Akasha Morgan.

48. Krippner et al., *Extraordinary Dreams*.

49. "Luke on Dreambridge," YouTube.

Bibliography

Burton, Tim. *Alice in Wonderland*. 2010; Burbank: Walt Disney Pictures, 2010. DVD.

De Blois, Dean, and Chris Sanders. *How to Train Your Dragon*. 2010; North Hollywood: Dreamworks Animated, 2014. DVD/Blu-ray.

The Discovery Channel. *The Power of Dreams, Part III: Sacred Sleep.* Silver Spring, MD: Discovery Communications, 1994. VHS.

Feinstein, David, and Stanley Krippner. *The Mythic Path*, 3rd ed. Santa Rosa, CA: Elite, 2006.

Foulkes, David. *Children's Dreaming and the Development of Consciousness.* Cambridge, MA: Harvard University Press, 1999.

Garfield, Patricia. *Your Child's Dreams.* New York: Ballantine Books, 1984.

Halonen, Arto. *A Dreamer and the Dream Tribe.* New York: Mystic Fire Video, 1998. VHS.

Hart, Tobin. *The Secret Spiritual World of Children.* Novato, CA: New World Library, 2003.

Jung, Carl G. *Memories, Dreams, Reflections.* Edited by Aniela Jaffé, trans. Richard and Clara Winston. New York: Vintage, 1989.

Kellogg, Ed. "Harry Potter and the Lucid Dream Exchange Challenge: Trying out Spells from the Hogwarts Universe." *The Lucid Dream Exchange* 24–26, no. 36, September 2005. Accessed December 12, 2005. http://www.dreaming lucid.com/using-magic-like-harry-potter/.

Krippner, Stanley, Fariba Bogzaran, and André Percia de Carvalho. *Extraordinary Dreams and How to Work with Them.* New York: SUNY Press, 2002.

Krippner, Stanley and Allan Combs. "Structures of Consciousness and Creativity: Opening the Doors of Perception." In *Everyday Creativity*, ed. Ruth Richards, 131–149. Washington, DC: APA, 2007.

Krippner, Stanley. "Anyone Who Dreams Partakes in Shamanism." *Journal of Shamanic Practice* 2, no. 2 (2009): 33–40.

Mallon, Brenda. *Dream Time with Children.* London: Jessica Kingsley, 2002.

Morgan, Angel K. "Luke on Dreambridge." YouTube video, 4:37. Posted June 23, 2013. https://www.youtube.com/watch?v=kGlf2I3VYlE.

Morgan, Angel K. "Dream Sharing as a Healing Method: Tropical Roots and Contemporary Community Potential." *Journal of Tropical Psychology* 4, no. 12 (2014): 1–16.

Morgan, Angel K. "Dreambridge Workshops & Courses." Accessed March 25, 2015. http://thedreambridge.com/workshops.htm.

Piaget, Jean. *The Psychology of the Child.* New York: Basic Books, 2000.

Staley, Betty. *Between Form and Freedom.* Stroud, UK: Hawthorn Press, 1988.

Steiner, Rudolf. *Education of the Child in the Light of Anthroposophy.* London: Rudolf Steiner Press, 1965.

Steiner, Rudolf. *The Kingdom of Childhood.* New York: Anthroposophic Press, 1995.

Steiner, Rudolf. *Education for Adolescents.* Barrington, MA: Anthroposophic Press, 1996.

Stewart, Kilton. "Mental Hygiene and World Peace." *Mental Hygiene* 38 (1954): 387–403.

Stewart, Kilton. "Dream Theory in Malaya." In *Altered States of Consciousness*, ed. Charles T. Tart, 161–170. New York: Doubleday, 1969.

Taylor, Jeremy. *Where People Fly and Water Runs Uphill.* New York: Warner Books, 1992.
Tedlock, Barbara. "Dreams." *Encyclopedia of Religion* 2nd ed., vol. 4, ed. L. Jones. Detroit, MI: Macmillan Reference USA (2005): 2482–2491.
Wachowksi, Andy, and Lana Wachowsky. *The Matrix.* Burbank: Warner Bros., 1999. DVD.

CHAPTER SIX

The Impact of Digital Technology on Children's Dreams

Jayne Gackenbach, Arielle Boyes, Ann Sinyard, Carson Flockhart, and Caterina Snyder

As part of Summer Art Camp, I asked the children to draw one of their most memorable, recent dreams. One boy (age 8) explained what he drew.

> *I am Darth Vader and I have a bright red lightsaber. Luke Skywalker wants to fight me. There are explosions all around me but I use the Force. I get into a spaceship and blast my way through the galaxy.*

As an afterthought he added: "I know that I am the bad guy, but I have lots of Storm Trooper friends," and that he liked to play *Star Wars: The Clone Wars* on his PlayStation.

This example illustrates how the role of video game play, and indeed electronic media, has become pervasive in today's society including in our dreams. By contrast, in the 1930s the average American child was exposed to approximately 10 hours of mass media *per week*. With the proliferation of technology in the twenty-first century, the average American child is now exposed to 10 hours and 45 minutes of mass media *per day*. Moreover, by 2010, 80 percent of children aged one to three regularly use the Internet.[1]

The Internet has changed the ways families interact. Today, it is not uncommon for families to gather around their Wii for a night of gaming or to see children occupied by tablet or cell phone games in waiting rooms to pass the time. New cars are commonly equipped with Internet and DVD players for backseat passengers. Some parents report feeling guilt over their child's online activities, fearing that media use has replaced other activities important for social development.[2] Infants and toddlers are developing digital footprints at younger ages than ever before with parents posting pregnancy pictures on social networking sites like Facebook before the child is even born. Parenting blogs are also on the rise. These blogs contain a variety of topics ranging from basic parenting advice to personal anecdotes of toilet training or child tantrums, parental frustrations, and photos of children.[3]

Like their parents, children are also using these new media. Initially, concerns focused primarily on the amount of television children watched. With the advent of interactive media, especially video game play, the attention turned to whether children should be playing video games and, if so, how much and which type was appropriate. As interactive media became an increasingly important part of our daily lives, the presence of video games in children's lives became increasingly accepted. Some proposed motivations for children's video game play include hanging out with friends, competition, making new friends, and leadership opportunities. Emotional motivations include regulating feelings or the mental state of being completely absorbed by a goal-drive task. For middle-school children, video game play may allow for a sense of challenge and mastery, creativity, and identity experimentation through the use of avatars or online profiles.[4]

In this chapter, we examine how media use is affecting children's lives. Given the continuity of dreams from waking life experiences, we will then consider how media use, and especially video game play, affects dreams.

How Does Technology Impact Children's Behaviors and Dreams?

> In a pre-kindergarten classroom located in a middle-class Midwestern city in the USA, . . . the children and teacher gathered . . . to explore . . . how dreams emerged and why they were so important. . . . "I dreamt I danced on my Wii with my sisters," responded Aleia. "I had a dream of playing my *Mario* game from when I wake up in the morning to when I go to bed at night."[5]

The increasingly important role of technology in nearly every aspect of children's lives undoubtedly affects not only their waking reality but also their perceived reality during sleep. Researchers and parents alike are concerned with understanding how exactly technology affects children and whether or not it is a positive or negative force in their lives.

The American Academy of Pediatrics' policy statement on media violence suggests that parents have reason for concern. Specifically, they posit that video games allow children to act out violence and they overgeneralize from the 1999 Columbine High School shootings as an example of video game play gone awry. According to the Academy, children exposed to media violence experience a range of health problems including aggressive behaviors, fear, violence, nightmares, and sleep disturbances.[6] While certainly there is concern when children are exposed to violence in any manner, the reaction to the Columbine shootings both in the press reports and by this professional society is essentially what one well-regarded gaming researcher noted as feeding a moral panic wheel. It is not based on systematic inquiry, in other words good science.

A comprehensive review of the research reveals a more complex relationship between children and digital technology. Some research suggests that children occasionally have nightmares based on television viewing or video game play,[7] but that dreams also help to regulate negative emotions.[8] Research on aggression and video game play, specifically, has found that multiple factors determine risk of aggression and that video game play does not cause violence universally but rather under specific circumstances or when used by a particular type of individual.[9] Thus, when we consider the role of media use in a child's life, and its impact on subsequent dreams, it is important to realize that it is neither the only nor the primary influence.

Nightmares and Technology

When queried about his three-year-old son's dreams regarding *Minecraft* video game play, Ryan Hurd wrote:

> I finally recalled one of Connor's exclamations about video games when waking up. One is a nightmare—the other one was not, apparently. Connor woke up crying and said, "A creeper just blew me up!" Another time he woke up and said (something like), "Daddy, pig zombies are nice."

These two dream segments from Connor illustrate the range of responses to gaming in dreams for children. A common stereotype is that video game play per se creates nightmares. While children may have nightmares they are likely not due to video game play. To say this is like saying that listening to radio creates nightmares, or reading a book creates nightmares, or watching TV creates nightmares. The nightmare comes as a function of the content of the media experience not the type of media engaged with.

A nightmare is defined as a distressing dream in which the dreamer is awakened from sleep with a recollection of the dream.[10] Both physiological and psychological stressors may predispose children to nightmares, since most nightmares are caused by and reflect the child's waking life. Traumatic events in particular, such as accidents, kidnappings, or rape, frequently lead to nightmares.[11] It is important to note, however, that nightmare frequency reports by parents and children are quite different, suggesting that parents are not always aware of their child's nightmares or that the child does not feel comfortable talking about them.[12] Needless to say, creating an open and welcoming dream dialogue in the household may lessen this effect.

One technology thought to directly impact dreaming, especially nightmares, is video games. Video games, especially violent video games, have been linked to some negative effects, including aggressive behavior and emotions; but when variables that we know contribute to aggression are controlled, then the effects are almost nonexistent. Furthermore, one unexpected positive benefit is that combat-centric video games may provide a sort of nightmare protection at least in late adolescence and adulthood. Researchers suggest that when a person plays a violent combat-centric game they may subsequently be able to avoid victimization in their dreams.[13] The protection effect, however, is only found in heavy gamers—that is, individuals who have spent thousands of hours gaming in their lifetime. Further, research suggests that the nightmare protection phenomena does not apply equally to both sexes and is generally found only in males and more masculine females in late adolescence.

One common finding across all studies, however, was that playing large amounts of combat-centric video games resulted in a decrease in threat experienced in nightmares. For instance, in a laboratory study run by Carson Flockhart on university freshmen, he reported on high-end gamers playing the combat-centric *Farcry* condition: "We saw dream reports such as 'In my dream I was a marine sniper, crawling through the bushes in a swamp.'" This fighting back was not present in those who played a non-combat game.

Another interesting finding of the nightmare protection research is that even if awakened by the dream, gamers are more likely to consider the "nightmare" as fun and perceive it like playing a combat-centric game. Gamers see a drastic change in their threat perception and reaction, and events or experiences that may paralyze others in dreams are instead an empowering challenge to overcome. In other words, heavy gamers experience dream events that bolster their confidence rather than create negative emotions, as illustrated by the following example:

> I was at a mall with a girl and everything was normal. All of a sudden, a large muscular man crashed through the ceiling and started killing innocent people. He claimed to be the prized creation of death himself, and was looking for a 'demon with wolf ears.' I changed into a werewolf and attacked the man.
>
> Jack, age 19

To non-gamers this dream might be both terrifying and paralyzing. The dreamer, however, was able to react quickly to the situation in a functional rather than fearful way. This effect derives from video game play as simulation where the dreamer is able to safely practice fighting back within a controlled context—the game.

The positive effect of video game play on nightmares suggests that video games may offer children a safe space in which to experiment with nightmare situations. Using dreams as a safe rehearsal ground for life's challenges is an evolutionary purpose for dreaming that researchers suggest in some ways mirrors the effect video games have on gamer's dreams.[14] Specifically, researchers theorized that dreams were paramount to our ancestor's survival because they allowed our brains to run simulations involving a myriad of threats and dangerous situations, which in turn improved our chances of survival should one of these situations arise. Video games, similarly, take the place of dream simulations and allow the dreamer to practice in the safe game space, subsequently increasing dreamer control and decreasing negative dream experiences. Children experiencing nightmares may benefit from some structured video game play with a parent in that it will help the child practice fighting back. Simulating the process of fighting back through video game play, however, may not be appropriate in all situations nor is it the beginning and end of the nightmare mediating effects associated with game play.

The content of children's dreams and nightmares has also been found to be affected by television watching. Jan Van den Bulck's study on first and fourth year Belgian elementary students found that while the children reported nightmare content related to computer game play, television content was also repeatedly featured.[15] Both boys and girls, however, reported pleasant dreams, which were frequently linked to both television and computer game content. In another study, Julia Stephan, Michael Schredl, Josie Henley-Einion, and Mark Blagrove examined the correlation between television viewing and nightmare frequency as well as self-rated effects of television content on dream content. The study researchers found that overall children's and adolescent's dream content is more affected by television than computer game play.[16] Parents are encouraged to participate in both video game play and television watching with their children so that they can discuss the experience.

Gaming, Lucid Dreaming, and Children

Various researchers have pointed out the similarities between video game play and lucid dreaming and in our laboratory at MacEwan we have found some statistical associations between gaming and lucidity in late adolescent students. Here is a dream example from 19-year-old Jakob:

> One of the earliest lucid dreams I can remember involved *Call of Duty* aspects. I was essentially in a nightmare being shot at with explosions all around me. I remember poking my head out to fire at the enemy when I noticed that I recognized the gun in my hands [and recognized it was a dream]. It was literally my favorite weapon from *Call of Duty*—an M16 rifle. . . . I leaped over the battlement and charged into what felt like familiarity. I knew which corners to look around as I entered the battle scarred rooms and there was constant destruction everywhere I went. There wasn't any fear embedded in me but an uncanny calm. I'm sure I was smiling in my sleep.

The idea that gaming may be a waking parallel to lucid dreaming is based on various parallels between these alternative realities. They are both more likely to be experienced and enjoyed due to the spatial skills of the dreamer. On a surface level the virtual worlds of gaming are similar to the biologically driven virtual world of the dream. In the latter case, if one knows it is a dream then the parallels become even stronger. Thus, while gamers report more lucid dreams than those who do not play, this has been an uneven finding in our laboratory. What has been consistent is the superiority of gamers to control subsequent dream content. This may or may not occur alongside lucidity. Sometimes gamers think that they are in a game while other times they think they are in a dream while asleep. The point is that in both cases they experience a sense of control over the dream/game. Here is a case of a young man in late adolescence, Fred, who had played Halo for several hours the day before this dream:

> I'm driving a car, again not at a real POV [point of view], but following behind the car. It didn't matter to me that I was crashing into other cars or walls. My car caught fire; I saw it melt from within. I died, not trying to escape.

When our team read this we assumed it was a lucid dream but we read on for his responses about the dream and Fred said it was not a lucid dream, but he did say that he noticed how the pixels were more obvious at various points. We then realized Fred thought he was in a game so it was OK to try dying in a fire! This is something one rarely finds in dreams or even in lucid dreams. Thus, this reality confusion among late adolescents and even adults is concerning.

Relatedly, David Oldis, a computer scientist and consultant with Dream Cloud, wrote recently in a personal communication about the potential of the new 3D goggles that are to be widely available from 2016. In this case he is referring to the Oculus Rift. He writes:

> I put the Rift on a three-year-old (the realistic "Tuscany Villa" program) and he was afraid because he was alone in the strange house, but afterward, wanted to go back "to the house *below* the table" (he was sitting at the table when he wore the Rift). I was ambivalent about even trying this, but children are already confronted with the mixed matrices of real, dream, game and media realities.
>
> So my thoughts on the future effect of VR [virtual reality] in our "matrix lives" are to examine this from a developmental perspective as one approach. How will the maturing brain and sense of self adjust to the revolving gallery of distinct "life worlds" each day—material, multiple VRs, dreams, media? From a phenomenological angle, what will "being" and "presence" become?

As provocative as the lucid dreaming potential is, it is not so easily generalized to preadolescent children as pointed out by Oldis. While there are ample anecdotal cases of lucidity in children, the problem is that reports of dreams from children are highly subject to demand characteristics of the inquiry. Children answer what they think the adult wants to hear. In addition, the very idea of knowing you are in a dream while still asleep can be hard for some adults to comprehend if they have never had the experience. It is considered to be a metacognitive skill in the lucid dreaming research literature. Such high levels of thinking about thinking are rare in children.

So the question may be: If my child plays video games will they then have more lucid dreams? We really do not know but there are a variety of improvements in attentional skills that can benefit them and perhaps one offshoot of that might be dreaming lucidly. While Barbra Wilson showed that most five-year-olds do perceive dreams as internal mental processes,[17] other researchers found that only 5 percent of children aged 10 years reported having lucid dreams, while 50 percent of 12- to 14-year-olds and 80–90 percent of 15- to 18-year-olds experienced lucid dreams.[18] These age differences in reports were also found in a 2012 study, by Ursula Voss, Clemens Frenzel, Judith Koppehele-Gossel, and Allan Hobson. This study revealed a steady trend of increased lucid dreaming from ages 6 to 13, where after age 13 the frequency of lucid dreams steadily declines.[19]

Video games, like fantasy and science fiction stories, also contain bizarre elements and may similarly affect the dreams of gamers and result in bizarre dreams. By definition, bizarre dreams contain content that is subjectively defined as strange.[20] Bizarreness is commonly found in the dreams and daydreams of adults with thin boundaries. Individuals with thick boundaries tend to make clear distinctions between different areas of their lives (e.g., work and play) whereas individuals with thin boundaries tend to be more open and make fewer distinctions.[21] As infants and toddlers, children demonstrate thin boundaries until they begin to thicken between the ages of 6 and 18.[22] Interestingly, bizarre dream content begins to increase around five to six years of age.[23] Heavy gamers, like young children and some adults, have been found to have thin boundaries. Accordingly, it may be that video games allow players to keep their boundaries thinner and subsequently open themselves up to both bizarre content and lucid dreams. The Gackenbach group has found associations between gaming, dream bizarreness, and lucidity.

Practical Tips for Parents

Children in the twenty-first century are growing up in an increasingly media rich world and their dreams and nightmares often reflect this changing reality. This in turn presents parents with a uniquely modern and sometimes seemingly overwhelming challenge to care for and support their children. Pediatric researchers and organizations offer a wide range of practical tips for parents, however, as well as evidence that their child's media consumption has not only negative but also positive side effects.

Parents can model positive media consumption behaviors and effective "media diets" to help their children learn to be selective and healthy in their media consumption. The Canadian Pediatrics Society suggests that the most comprehensive way to get involved with the child's media use is by watching, playing, listening, and talking with the child.[24] For example, parents can become more involved in their child's TV watching and gaming by using new technology (TiVo, DVR, DVDs, online videos, etc.) to pause the program and discuss what they are seeing. The American Academy of Pediatrics further suggests making a Family Media Use Plan that creates rules surrounding media use.[25] An example of this would be allowing media use in the house (TV, cell phones, and Internet) only after children have completed their homework. They also suggest that parents limit their child's media consumption to one or two hours per day and that children younger than two have minimal or no screen media exposure.

In addition, parents are encouraged to create a strong bedtime routine; keeping screens out of children's bedrooms and limiting screen time immediately before bed, due to its disruptive influence on sleep.[26] It has been found that adolescents who spend large amounts of time using electronic devices during either the day or night have an increased risk of short sleep duration, long time to fall asleep, and increased need for sleep.

Another way parents can play a more active role in their children's media consumption is to educate themselves on the rating system of that specific media. The video game industry, for example, has an Entertainment Software Ratings Board (ESRB) rating for almost every game produced and gaming consoles themselves have embedded parental control tools. These tools allow parents to enter the ESRB rating level that they believe is acceptable for their children to play. Once they do so, no game rated above that level can be played on the console.[27] Parents should focus not only on standard rating systems but also on:

- knowing more about the media their child consumes;
- knowing how and when their child consumes media;
- what their child is sensitive to;
- what their family values are.

Finally, encouraging new and different types of entertainment (e.g., hiking) also help children make good choices when faced with a decision between a sedentary media-based lifestyle versus a more active and engaged one. Encouraging good media and active living habits when children are young, in particular, is paramount because as children age it becomes harder to enforce limits and influence their choices. Ultimately, what is needed for children to flourish is a strong balance between media consumption and other forms of entertainment.

The Positive Effects of Digital Media

Although heavy media use in children and adolescents may cause some negative side effects, it is also associated with positive developments. Virtual Reality Exposure Therapy, for example, uses video games to combat a variety of anxiety disorders, phobias, and public speaking fears, as well as post-traumatic stress disorder (PTSD). In one study of active duty soldiers, seeking treatment following a deployment resulted in a significant reduction of PTSD symptoms after using the virtual reality game (i.e., *Virtual Iraq*).[28] Other medical uses for video game therapy are being explored including using games to treat attention deficit hyperactivity disorder (ADHD), Alzheimer's, schizophrenia, asthma, motor rehabilitation, impulse-related disorders,[29] and burn victim recovery.[30] Although both video game therapy and virtual reality exposure therapy are currently in the early development stages, they offer a potentially unique treatment solution for a wide range of conditions, including nightmares.

Researchers have explored the relationship between creativity, which facilitates the development of new ideas, and video game play. In a 2012 study of young adolescents, researchers found that video game play was associated with creativity while other forms of media, such as computers, Internet, and cell phones, were not.[31] Other studies, conversely, have not found a relationship between creativity and video game play. In a study of fourth and fifth graders, researcher Karla Hamlen[32] found no connection between gaming and creativity. Researchers Jayne Gackenbach and Raelyne Dopko, in contrast, found a positive relationship between video game play and spatial creativity, if not verbal creativity, among late adolescent college students.

Although the relationship between creativity and media use, including gaming, appears to be mixed, some children's creativity is clearly affected by gaming. For instance, one of this chapter's authors shares her own experience with gaming and creativity as a child:

> The students, myself included, of my 1996 grade one class were exposed to computers on a regular basis. We were to complete modules teaching us to type. If we finished early, we were allowed to play computer games such as *Storybook Weaver*. *Storybook Weaver* allowed users to interactively design pictures and then write stories based on these pictures. My time spent building stories based on these computer programs is one of the only things I remember of grade one.

Minecraft, similar to *Storybook Weaver*, is a video game that falls into the unique category of creative gaming. The purpose of the *Minecraft* is to allow players to exercise their creativity in a universe made of Lego blocks, where gamers can do whatever they want with the environment. They can build houses or castles and some people have done full-scale paintings using the small blocks and pixels. This open world, or "sand-box" genre, allows gamers endless creativity and, unsurprisingly, affects their dreams.

In addition to potentially bolstering creativity, video games have been found to show other positive effects. Specifically, video game play may increase certain cognitive faculties, which have wide reaching implications for today's youth. These effects are strongest in high action games. In particular, research has shown that children who play first person shooter games improved their attention allocation, spatial resolution of visual processing, and mental rotation abilities. These increases in cognitive ability have been shown to be equivalent to those seen from university level courses promoting the same skills. Furthermore, these spatial skills develop quickly and last over an extended period of time. The improvements also transfer to skills outside of the gaming context. Consequently, developing improved spatial skills may help youth interested in science or mathematics excel and have even been linked to repeated long-term career success.[33]

While video games have been shown to increase attention and visual motor and spatial skills, they may have other real world applications as well. Some research has found that playing high action games resulted in a transfer of learning effect. This suggests that game play appeared to increase participants' ability to learn new tasks. In short, playing high action video games improved the learning transfer.[34] Here is an example from a young hockey player who spoke of starting to play at age eight and how gaming informed his real world hockey play. Jakob writes:

> Competition was always something I was fond of as a child. One of my main draws to the sport of hockey was just that. It was a fight in the rink, with victors and losers. I remember one reason that I chose to be a goaltender was that the intensity of the game rested on your shoulders. ... This tied into my video game play as I was heavily invested in the outcomes of the first person shooters. ... I noticed that when I began playing video games more consistently, my reflexes and reactions to things were much more affluent. In the game of hockey I was able to keep track of the entire five-man team effectively, as well as track the speedy puck as it moved around during the play. Now I note that my many years of hockey allowed me to gain the skills I did on the ice, however I truly believe that my hours clocked playing video games assisted me and took me to the next level.

Probably one of the most interesting and important findings regarding gaming for all ages is that it helps to manage the mental chatter that can be so stressful. This ranges from simple distraction to full promotion of the meditative relaxation response.[35] Carmen Russoniello, of East Carolina University, is at the forefront of the research on casual games and their relaxing benefits. Russoniello was approached by a major game developer to explore why their games were selling so well. What he discovered is that on a psychological, as well as physiological level, casual video game play produces the same relaxation response found in meditation. But so, too, do the more action-centered games offer aid in mental fixation. A young African college student, Fred, writes of his experience regarding a profound loss of faith:

> The existential crisis I experienced worried me greatly, and thoughts of dying, nihilistic thoughts of not having a purpose at all, and feelings of helplessness pervaded my thoughts at all hours of the day no matter how hard I tried to suppress them ... where I would find the closest thing to solace was when I would play immersive video games like *Mass Effect* where technologically constructed alternative realities drew in the player, demanded undivided attention and cultivated absorption.

But it was his experiences at night that are especially provocative:

> I would lie in bed (where my distress would be at its peak), pondering rest-
> lessly about death and mortality, unable to relax, and then find myself
> experiencing awful variations of a dream where my eyes fade to black and
> I enter a purgatory-like state ... I would sometimes, mercifully, become
> aware that I was simply experiencing a nightmare, and instead of waking
> up ... I would think of *Mass Effect* scenarios such as walking through the
> "citadel" map, firing assault rifles and taking cover with allies—basically
> implanting myself in the fictional reality ... and my sense of comfort and
> calm was almost normal. I knew I was dreaming because I would remind
> myself not to get overzealous and "wake up."

Other students at our university have testified about how playing a very
absorbing video game helped in recovery from major depression. Kyle writes:

> During my grade 11 year ... I found myself spiraling out of control, starting
> with my own mother's diagnosis of being depressed, mixed with the unrelent-
> ing course load. I found myself slipping deep down into the dark mental trap
> known as depression. It consumed me for more than 9 months, leaving me
> with absolutely no will to do anything, lying on a couch watching TV. Then
> one day I was coaxed out of the house by my dad to go to a computer shop
> to help him get some software and I saw *World of Warcraft* (*WoW*) on the shelf.

He became a dedicated *WoW* player and concludes, "Through a combination
of being a guilt leader, master of my characters, and the aid provided by my
doctor I managed a full recovery." In this age of the dominance of cognitive
behavioral therapies especially for the escalating epidemic of depression
among college students, gaming offers an intuitive and easy intervention.

Notes

1. Aviva Lucas Gutnick et al., *Always Connected: The New Digital Media Habits of Young Children* (New York: The Joan Ganz Cooney Center at Sesame Workshop, 2010), accessed October 26, 2015, http://www.joanganzcooneycenter.org/wp -content/uploads/2011/03/jgcc_alwaysconnected.pdf.

2. Alexis Lauricella et al., "Parenting in the Age of Technology: Parent Attitudes and Behaviors Related to Children's Media Use" (Presentation, Annual Meeting of the International Communication Association, Hilton Metropole Hotel, London, England, June 17, 2014).

3. Dublin Institute of Technology (DIT), "Remember Toddler Privacy Online," *Science Daily*, accessed September 22, 2013, http://www.sciencedaily.com/releases/ 2013/09/130902123916.htm.

4. Cheryl K. Olson, "Children's Motivations for Video Game Play in the Context of Normal Development," *Review of General Psychology* 14, no. 2 (2010): 180–187, doi: 10.1037/a0018984.

5. Kathleen Harris, "Teacher, I Had a Dream: A Glimpse of the Spiritual Domain of Children Using Project-Based Learning," *International Journal of Children's Spirituality* 18, no. 3 (2013): 281–293, doi: 10.1080/1364436X.2013.858665.

6. Council on Communications and Media, "Policy Statement—Media Violence," *Pediatrics* 124, no. 5 (2009):1495–1503, doi: 10.1542/peds.2009-2146.

7. Frederick Zimmerman, "Children's Media Use and Sleep Problems: Issues and Unanswered Questions," *Kaiser Family Foundation* (2008), https://kaiserfamilyfoundation.files.wordpress.com/2013/01/7674.pdf.

8. Ross Levin and Tore Nielsen, "Nightmares, Bad Dreams, and Emotional Dysregulation: A Review and New Neurocognitive Model of Dreaming," *Current Directions in Psychological Science* 18, no. 2 (2009): 84–88, doi: 10.1111/j.1467-8721.2009.01614.x.

9. Patrick M. Markey and Charlotte N. Markey, "Vulnerability to Violent Video Games: A Review and Integration of Personality Research," *Review of General Psychology* 14, no. 2 (2010): 82–91, doi: http://dx.doi.org/10.1037/a0019000.

10. Mark Blagrove, Laura Farmer, and Elvira Williams, "The Relationship of Nightmare Frequency and Nightmare Distress to Well-Being," *Journal of Sleep Research* 13, no. 2 (2004): 129–136, doi: 10.1111/j.1365-2869.2004.00394.x.

11. Alexander K. C. Leung and William Lane M. Robson, "Nightmares," *Journal of the National Medical Association* 85, no. 3 (1993): 233–235, PMC2571879.

12. Michael Schredl et al., "Factors Affecting Nightmares in Children: Parents' vs. Children's Ratings," *European Child & Adolescent Psychiatry* 18, no. 1 (2009): 20–25, doi:10.1007/s00787-008-0697-5.

13. All references to the work in Jayne Gackenbach's laboratory at MacEwan University can be found in: Johnathan Bown and Jayne Gackenbach, "Video Games, Nightmares, and Emotional Processing," in *Emotions and Technology: Communication of Feelings through, with and for Technology*, ed. S. Tettegah (London: Elsevier, Academic Psychology Division, 2015).

14. Katja Valli et al., "The Threat Simulation Theory of the Evolutionary Function of Dreaming: Evidence from Dreams of Traumatized Children," *Consciousness and Cognition* 14, no. 1 (2005): 188–218, doi:10.1016/S1053-8100(03)00019-9.

15. Jan Van den Bulck, "Media Use and Dreaming: The Relationship among Television Viewing, Computer Game Play and Nightmares or Pleasant Dreams," *Dreaming* 14, no. 1 (2004): 43–49, doi: HYPERLINK "http://psycnet.apa.org/doi/10.1037/1053-0797.14.1.43" \t "_blank"10.1037/1053-0797.14.1.43.

16. Julia Stephan et al., "TV Viewing and Dreaming in Children: The UK Library Study," *International Journal of Dream Research* 5, no. 2 (2012): 130–133, doi: http://dx.doi.org/10.11588/ijodr.2012.2.9454.

17. Barbra J. Wilson, "Children's Reaction to Dreams Conveyed on Mass Media Programming," *Communication Research* 18 (1991): 283–305, doi: 10.1177/009365091018003001.

18. N. Lapina, V. Lysenko, and A. Burikov, "Age-Dependent Dreaming: Characteristics of Secondary School Pupils," *Sleep Supplement* 21 (1998): 287.

19. Ursula Voss et al., "Lucid Dreaming: An Age-Dependent Brain Dissociation," *Journal of Sleep Research* 21, no. 6 (2012): 634–642, doi: 10.1111/j.1365-2869.2012.01022.x.

20. Nirit Soffer-Dudek and Avi Sadeh."Dream Recall Frequency and Unusual Dream Experiences in Early Adolescence: Longitudinal Links to Behavior Problems," *Journal of Research on Adolescence* 23, no. 4 (2013): 635–651. DOI: 10.1111/jora.12007.

21. Robert Kunzendorf et al., "Bizarreness of the Dreams and Daydreams Reported by Individuals with Thin and Thick Boundaries,"*Dreaming* 7, no. 4 (1997): 265–271, doi: http://dx.doi.org/10.1037/h0094482.

22. Ernest Hartmann and Robert Kunzendorf, "The Central Image (CI) in Recent Dreams, Dreams That Stand Out, and Earliest Dreams: Relationship to Boundaries," *Imagination, Cognition, and Personality* 25, no. 4 (2006):383–392, doi: 10.2190/0Q56-1445-3J16-3831.

23. Claudio Colace, "Children's Dreaming: A Study Based on Questionnaires Completed by Parents," *Sleep and Hypnosis* 8, no. 1 (2006): 19–32, retrieved from http://www.sleepandhypnosis.org/pdf/8_1_4.pdf.

24. Canadian Paediatric Society, "Caring for Kids," June 1, 2011, accessed October 27, 2015, http://www.caringforkids.cps.ca/handouts/limiting_screen_time_at_home.

25. American Academy of Pediatrics, "Managing Media: We Need a Plan," October 28, 2013, accessed October 27, 2015, https://www.aap.org/en-us/about-the-aap/aap-press-room/pages/Managing-Media-We-Need-a-Plan.aspx.

26. Mari Hysing et al., "Sleep and Use of Electronic Devices in Adolescence: Results from a Large Population-Based Study," *BMJ Open* 5, no. 1 (2015): 1–7, doi: 10.1136/bmjopen-2014-006748.

27. Entertainment Software Ratings Board, "ESRB Ratings Guide," accessed October 27, 2015, https://www.esrb.org/ratings/ratings_guide.aspx.

28. Maryrose Gerardi et al., "Virtual Reality Exposure Therapy Using a Virtual Iraq: Case Report," *Journal of Traumatic Stress* 21, no. 2 (2008): 209–213, doi: 10.1002/jts.20331.

29. Fernando Fernández-Aranda et al., "Video Games as a Complementary Therapy Tool in Mental Disorders: PlayMancer, a European Multicenter Study," *Journal of Mental Health* 21, no. 4 (2012): 364–374, doi: 10.3109/09638237.2012.664302.

30. Hunter G. Hoffman et al., "Feasibility of Articulated Arm Mounted Oculus Rift Virtual Reality Goggles for Adjunctive Pain Control During Occupational Therapy in Pediatric Burn Patients," *Cyberpsychology, Behavior and Social Networking* 17, no. 6 (2014): 397–401, doi: 10.1089/cyber.2014.0058.

31. Linda A. Jackson et al. "Information Technology Use and Creativity: Findings from the Children and Technology Project," *Computers in Human Behavior* 28, no. 2 (2012): 370–376, doi: 10.1016/j.chb.2011.10.006.

32. Karla Hamlen, "Relationships Between Computer and Video Game Play and Creativity Among Upper Elementary School Students," *Journal of Educational Computing Research* 40, no. 1 (2009): 1–21, doi: 10.2190/EC.40.1.a.

33. Isabela Granic, Adam Lobel, and C.M.E. Rutger, "The Benefits of Playing Video Games," *American Psychologist* 69, no. 1 (2014): 66–78, doi: http://dx.doi.org/10.1037/a0034857.

34. C. S. Green and D. Bavelier, "Learning, Attention and Action Video Games," *Current Biology* 22, no. 6 (2012): 197–206, doi: 10.1016/j.cub.2012.02.012.

35. C. Russoniello, K. O'Brien, and J. Parks, "The Effectiveness of Casual Video Games in Improving Mood and Decreasing Stress," *Journal of Cyber Therapy & Rehabilitation* 2, no. 1 (2009): 53–66.

Bibliography

American Academy of Pediatrics. "Managing Media: We Need a Plan." October 28, 2013. Accessed October 27, 2013. https://www.aap.org/en-us/about-the-aap/aap-press-room/pages/Managing-Media-We-Need-a-Plan.aspx.

Blagrove, Mark, Farmer, Laura and Williams, Elvira."The Relationship of Nightmare Frequency and Nightmare Distress to Well-Being." *Journal of Sleep Research* 13, no. 2 (2004): 129–136. doi: 10.1111/j.1365-2869.2004.00394.x.

Bown, Johnathan and Jayne Gackenbach. "Video Games, Nightmares, and Emotional Processing." In *Emotions and Technology: Communication of Feelings through, with and for Technology*, ed. S. Tettegah. (London: Elsevier, Academic Psychology Division, 2015).

Canadian Paediatric Society. "Caring For Kids." June 1, 2011. Accessed October 27, 2015. http://www.caringforkids.cps.ca/handouts/limiting_screen_time_at_home.

Colace, Claudio. "Children's Dreaming: A Study Based on Questionnaires Completed by Parents." *Sleep and Hypnosis* 8, no. 1 (2006): 19–32. Accessed October 27, 2015. http://www.sleepandhypnosis.org/pdf/8_1_4.pdf.

Council on Communications and Media. "Policy Statement—Media Violence." *Pediatrics* 124, no. 5 (2009): 1495–1503. doi: 10.1542/peds.2009-2146.

Dublin Institute of Technology (DIT). "Remember Toddler Privacy Online." *Science Daily*. Accessed September 22, 2013. http://www.sciencedaily.com/releases/2013/09/130902123916.htm.

Entertainment Software Rating Board. "ESRB Ratings Guide." Accessed October 27, 2015. https://www.esrb.org/ratings/ratings_guide.jsp.

Fernández-Aranda, Fernando, Susana Jiménez-Murcia, Juan J. Santamaría, Katarina Gunnard, Antonio Soto, Elias Kalapanidas, Richard G. Bults, Costas Davarakis, Todor Ganchev, Roser Granero, Dimitri Konstantas, Theodoros P. Kostoulas, Tony Lam, Mikkel Lucas, Cristina Masuet-Aumatell, Maher H. Moussa, Jeppe Nielsen, and Eva Penelo. "Video Games as a Complementary Therapy Tool in Mental Disorders: PlayMancer, a European Multicenter

Study." *Journal of Mental Health* 21, no. 4 (2012): 364–374. doi: 10.3109/09638237.2012.664302.

Gerardi, Maryrose, Barbara Olasov Rothbaum, Kerry Ressler, Mary Heekin, and Albert Rizzo. "Virtual Reality Exposure Therapy Using a Virtual Iraq: Case Report."*Journal of Traumatic Stress* 21, no. 2 (2008): 209–213. doi: 10.1002/jts.20331.

Granic, Isabela, Adam Lobel, and , C.M.E. Rutger. "The Benefits of Playing Video Games." *American Psychologist* 69, no. 1 (2014): 66–78. doi: http://dx.doi.org/10.1037/a0034857.

Green, C. S. and D. Bavelier. "Learning, Attention and Action Video Games." *Current Biology* 22, no. 6 (2012): 197–206. doi:10.1016/j.cub.2012.02.012.

Gutnick, Aviva Lucas, Michael Robb, Lori Takeuchi, and Jennifer Kotler. *Always Connected: The New Digital Media Habits of Young Children.* New York: The Joan Ganz Cooney Center at Sesame Workshop, 2010. Accessed October 26, 2015. http://www.joanganzcooneycenter.org/wp-content/uploads/2011/03/jgcc_always connected.pdf.

Hamlen, Karla. "Relationships between Computer and Video Game Play and Creativity among Upper Elementary School Students." *Journal of Educational Computing Research* 40, no. 1 (2009): 1–21. doi: 10.2190/EC.40.1.a.

Harris, Kathleen. "Teacher, I Had a Dream: A Glimpse of the Spiritual Domain of Children Using Project-Based Learning." *International Journal of Children's Spirituality* 18, no. 3 (2013): 281–293. doi: 10.1080/1364436X.2013.858665.

Hartmann, Ernest and Robert Kunzendorf. "The Central Image (CI) in Recent Dreams, Dreams That Stand Out, and Earliest Dreams: Relationship to Boundaries." *Imagination, Cognition, and Personality* 25, no. 4 (2006): 383–392. doi: 10.2190/0Q56-1445-3J16-3831.

Hoffman, Hunter G., Walter J. Meyer, Maribel Ramirez, Linda Roberts, Eric J. Seibel, Barbara Atzori, Sam R. Sharar, R. Sam, and David R. Patterson. "Feasibility of Articulated Arm Mounted Oculus Rift Virtual Reality Goggles for Adjunctive Pain Control during Occupational Therapy in Pediatric Burn Patients." *Cyberpsychology, Behavior and Social Networking* 17, no. 6 (2014): 397–401. doi:10.1089/cyber.2014.0058.

Hysing, Mari, Ståle Pallesen, Kjell Morten Stormark, Reidar Jakobsen, Astri J. Lundervold, and Børge Sivertsen. "Sleep and Use of Electronic Devices in Adolescence: Results from a Large Population-Based Study." *BMJ Open* 5, no. 1 (2015): 1–7. doi: 10.1136/bmjopen-2014-006748.

Jackson, Linda A., Edward A. Witt, Alexander Ivan Games, Hiram E. Fitzgerald, Alexander von Eye, and Yong Zhao. "Information Technology Use and Creativity: Findings from the Children and Technology Project." *Computers in Human Behaviour* 28, no. 2 (2012): 370–376. doi:10.1016/j.chb.2011.10.006.

Kunzendorf, Robert, Ernest Hartmann, Rachel Cohen, and Jennifer Cutler."Bizarreness of the Dreams and Daydreams Reported by Individuals with Thin and Thick Boundaries." *Dreaming* 7, no. 4 (1997): 265–271.doi: http://dx.doi.org/10.1037/h0094482.

Lapina, N., V. Lysenko, and A. Burikov. "Age-Dependent Dreaming: Characteristics of Secondary School Pupils." *Sleep Supplement* 21 (1998): 287.

Lauricella, Alexis, Ariel Maschke, Sabrina Connell, Ellen Wartella, and Victoria Rideout. "Parenting in the Age of Technology: Parent Attitudes and Behaviors Related to Children's Media Use." Presentation, Annual Meeting of the International Communication Association, Hilton Metropole Hotel, London, England, June 17, 2014. Retrieved from: http://citation.allacademic.com/meta/p632171_index.html.

Leung, Alexander K. C. and William Lane M. Robson. "Nightmares." *Journal of the National Medical Association* 85, no. 3 (1993): 233–235. PMC2571879.

Levin, Ross and Tore Nielsen. "Nightmares, Bad Dreams, and Emotional Dysregulation: A Review and New Neurocognitive Model of Dreaming." *Current Directions in Psychological Science* 18, no. 2 (2009): 84–88. doi: 10.1111/j.1467-8721.2009.01614.x.

Markey, Patrick M. and Charlotte N. Markey. "Vulnerability to Violent Video Games: A Review and Integration of Personality Research." *Review of General Psychology* 14, no. 2 (2010): 82–91. doi: http://dx.doi.org/10.1037/a0019000.

Olson, Cheryl K. "Children's Motivations for Video Game Play in the Context of Normal Development." *Review of General Psychology* 14, no. 2 (2010): 180–187. doi: 10.1037/a0018984.

Piaget, Jean. "*Weltbild des Kindes—Kapitel 3: Die Träume.*" Stuttgart: Klett-Cotta, 1978.

Russoniello, C., K. O'Brien, and J. Parks. "The Effectiveness of Casual Video Games in Improving Mood and Decreasing Stress." *Journal of Cyber Therapy & Rehabilitation* 2, no. 1 (2009): 53–66.

Schredl, Michael, Leonie Fricke-Oerkermann, Alexander Mitschke, Alfred Wiater, and Gerd Lehmkuhl. "Factors Affecting Nightmares in Children: Parents' vs. Children's Ratings." *European Child & Adolescent Psychiatry* 18, no. 1 (2009): 20–25. doi:10.1007/s00787-008-0697-5.

Soffer-Dudek, Nirit and Avi Sadeh. "Dream Recall Frequency and Unusual Dream Experiences in Early Adolescence: Longitudinal Links to Behavior Problems." *Journal of Research on Adolescence* 23, no. 4 (2013): 635–651. doi: 10.1111/jora.12007.

Stephan, Julia, Michael Schredl, Josie Henley-Einion, and Mark Blagrove. "TV Viewing and Dreaming in Children: The UK Library Study." *International Journal of Dream Research* 5, no. 2 (2012): 130–133. doi: http://dx.doi.org/10.11588/ijodr.2012.2.9454.

Valli, Katja, Antti Revonsuo, Outi Palkas, Ismail Hassan, Ali Kamaran, Karzan Jalal, and Raija-Leena Punamaki. "The Threat Simulation Theory of the Evolutionary Function of Dreaming: Evidence from Dreams of Traumatized Children." *Consciousness and Cognition* 14, no. 1 (2005): 188–218. doi:10.1016/S1053-8100(03)00019-9.

Van den Bulck, Jan. "Media Use and Dreaming: The Relationship among Television Viewing, Computer Game Play and Nightmares or Pleasant Dreams." *Dreaming* 14, no. 1 (2004): 43–49. doi: 10.1037/1053-0797.14.1.43.

Voss, Ursula, C. Frenzel, J. Koppehele-Gossel, and A. Hobson. "Lucid Dreaming: An Age-Dependent Brain Dissociation." *Journal of Sleep Research* 21, no. 6 (2012): 634–642. doi: 10.1111/j.1365-2869.2012.01022.x.

Wilson, Barbra J. "Children's Reaction to Dreams Conveyed on Mass Media Programming." *Communication Research* 18 (1991): 283–305. doi: 10.1177/009365091018003001.

Zimmerman, Frederick. "Children's Media Use and Sleep Problems: Issues and Unanswered Questions." *Kaiser Family Foundation.* 2008. https://kaiserfamily foundation.files.wordpress.com/2013/01/7674.pdf.

CHAPTER SEVEN

The Influence of Community on Children's Dreams

Martha A. Taylor

I dreamed I was a magic fluffy marshmallow jumping on the clouds. I had a smiley marshmallow face and the sky was blue.

Amelia, age 8

The diversity of the circles in which our children grow has an impact on them and on their dreams. How this might circle around to affect the community is significant to us in our lives and in our world. In this chapter, I will explore the community context as it relates to children's dreams. What happens to us as children is very influential in shaping who we become and in growing our best self. In the following story I share what began a lifelong love and interest in the well-being and health of children, all from a dream that grew in me.

When I was a small child, I often watched my father getting ready to go out somewhere, and I would always ask him, "Where are you going, Daddy?" He would invariably say, "I'm going to Timbuktu. Want to come along?" Of course, I would say "yes," not knowing where that was. If he was going, I wanted to be with him. As I grew older, my curiosity about Timbuktu stayed with me. I discovered that it was in Africa, and I read all I could about this mysterious country. Later as a young adult with a nursing license, I had an opportunity to travel to Uganda, East Africa, to take the place of another nurse who wanted to study in the United States. I was assigned to work with children in a small hospital in a remote village where I experienced seeing diseases I had only read about in the United States.

One day, a 13-year-old mother brought in her five-day-old baby boy saying; "He will not suck"—that is, she could not get the baby to nurse. As I touched him, he began to convulse. In the village they think mud will heal the umbilical cord. This tiny baby had tetanus, coming from the dirt used to treat the now infected cord. In order to treat this very lethal disease, the mother must not hold her child, who needs to lie very still to keep him from convulsing. With no common language, this young mother and I bonded to save her baby, her first child. He kept holding on to life in spite of death hovering very near. He was being fed through a tube, receiving strong medication, getting pneumonia, and not being able to move his very stiff muscles.

For a month, his mother stayed by his side day and night. One day she asked about his bowels. He had not passed stool. I suggested she wait a few more days. But in the morning I found her sitting on the floor with the baby's bottom up on her lap. She had one end of a reed in his bottom and the other end in her mouth giving him an enema. How does a mother just know? The baby moved his bowels, and began to improve steadily. A few months later, when he was past the worst, I told her to take him home and continue to exercise his very stiff muscles. More than a year later she came walking all the way from her home in the Congo (across the border from Uganda). She came to show me her healthy son and to thank me. This simple expression opened my desire to care for children for the rest of my life.

I share my childhood story because it shows how something seemingly simple between a young child and her father can impact one's whole life. The experience of living within this African village showed me the importance community played in my own development and in my future career.

The Community as Context for Children's Dreams

Research and my own experience show how much we can impact the lives of those around us by learning more about dreams. Dreams can teach us about ourselves, about our children, and about our world. They can give us practice in dealing with the big issues of our lives. Here I explore how children's dreams influence the world around them through their own community.

What does community mean when we speak about it as context? Children are born into a particular place from which they evolve. We are all born into some form of community. Some are born into poverty and some into riches, some in between. Some of us have the opportunity to have brothers and sisters and two loving parents. These circumstances are as diverse as the people we will become as we grow up in our particular milieu.

The word *community* has many diverse definitions depending on one's orientation. A community can be a social group, like a gathering of neighbors, or the group of friends our children go to school or play with. It can refer to a town or suburb. The word *community* can refer to shared common interests that might distinguish one group from other groups in our culture. For example, our children might go to a religious school or even a private school that has certain common values. The place where we work has distinguishing characteristics from any other workplace. It could be a religious group that has particular values. For a scientist, community can mean a group of organisms or populations living and interacting with one another in a particular environment. These organisms affect each other's abundance and their evolutionary adaptation. Depending on how broadly one views the interaction between organisms, a community can be small and local, as in a pond or tree; or regional or global, as in a biome.

In community, we come together with a group of individuals in a common desire to build something bigger and better than we might do as individuals alone. Community can be as small as the person I am most connected to in my life and as large as a global effort working to create a cleaner environment. It must include broad categories such as politics, economics, and all our social circles because these all strongly influence us in living out our dreams. We take what we value as individuals and find our own way to develop it by gathering others around us who share these values. We say "no man is an island" out of the belief that we are better and stronger with the bonds that bind us to each other.

We often speak of our "family tree." We have ancestors, grandparents, and parents and perhaps siblings. We are rooted in the soil of those who came before us. We might be the youngest, oldest, or middle child. We have a particular personality and interests. Dreams can help us learn about aspects that we might not yet be conscious of in our daily life. Once children branch out from parents, they develop many of their own influences. Their circles will include the type of schooling, homeschooling, or nonschooling they receive as well as what friends they make, what neighbors they play with, and what kind of parenting they receive. We might learn from their dreams something of the impact these have on their daily joys and stresses. Research shows that dreams evolve beginning in childhood. The dreams of young children are simpler and increase in complexity as they develop.[1]

The Value of Telling Dreams

> When you consider the plasticity of the brain—with as little as 10–12 minutes
> of motor practice a day on a specific task (say, piano playing) the motor cortex
> reshapes itself in a matter of a few weeks—the time spent in our dreams would
> surely shape how our brains develop, and influence our future behavioral pre-
> dispositions. The experiences we accrue from dreaming across our life span are
> sure to influence how we interact with the world and are bound to influence
> our overall fitness, not only as individuals but as a species.[2]

Jonathan Gottschalk refers to night dreams using the term *night stories*.
He shows us what an influence dreaming has in our behavior and our very
evolution as a species.

We learn from research that "telling dreams to other persons is more
likely if feelings of closeness, trust and understanding already exist in the
relationship and that telling dreams enhances closeness to the other person."[3] Children tend to pick their mothers as their closest connection in
sharing dreams.[4]

I only began to notice my own dreams during my transition into adulthood. However, I had made a career out of caring for and about children,
so when I recently read about Jill Gregory's experience teaching a children's
class on dreams, I was very interested. She noted:

> When I reflect on what a difference it would have made to me in my life to
> have had that wonderful resource (i.e., dreams) accessible, I've wanted so
> much to offer that gift to children. But I always assumed that a public school
> would never consider permitting dreams in the classroom, so I focused my
> energies on opening the dream-world to my own two children and their
> friends who visited our home.[5]

What Gregory discovered when she actually found a place open to
teaching children about dreams was that "most of all, they were literally
desperate to share their own dreams, hear some of my dreams and get
answers to their questions about dreams."[6] My own experience confirms
these words.

Dreams at Blue Mountain School

I wanted to see if I could help children become more aware of and helped
by their dreams and the dreams of their classmates. I live in a small town in
southwest Virginia. It is an artistic community with many potters,

musicians, and lively dances on a Friday night at the Country Store. It has deeply ingrained religious traditions. Many locals have been farmers for generations raising cows, chickens, and a variety of other crops.

I had been volunteering with a class of 8- to 10-year-olds in a small alternative school in town. This class had 11 students: 4 boys and 7 girls. They were a group that loved to talk and enjoyed holding one another's attention. Many had been together since they started school. They seemed very friendly with each other and considerate in their interactions. Their parents tended to be interested in a more open style of education, which was offered at this school. They wanted to encourage diversity and learning "outside the box." This model of education used many games and art projects for learning math and reading skills, which the kids explored with enthusiasm. During my first year with them, I observed they had a close connection with each other and with their wonderful Montessori teacher. I had previously shared many stories of my travels in other countries, and helped them with their studies four days a week. So we were already comfortable with each other.

I received approval to teach this class from the principal, who already knew me as a volunteer. They gave me a time during the last month of school that year as an experiment. This school uses a method of education called "contemplative progressive" that has evolved over the past 30 years since the school began as a place for the children of parents disillusioned with traditional schools. It views learning as a social venture that takes place through relationship. Although the learning style uses a curriculum map, it attempts to develop skills that are based on research into child development.[7]

Working with Dreams in the Classroom

As we began, I imagined that these students were my children and we were going on a trip together. First, they would need to prepare. Preparation in a classroom meant moving around and letting off steam. I developed a transition with music, songs, and movement. We then gathered in a circle on the floor. They needed to know where we were going: on a journey into the nighttime to see what we could find there. What are dreams and where do they come from? How can we remember them? What can they teach us? We began to pack our bags by exploring these questions. Most students remembered dreams occasionally, with only one of the boys saying he never dreamed. Dreams, they thought, were stories about vacations, or very frightening ones with monsters and zombies. There were magical and fun things, and sometimes you knew you were dreaming while you were dreaming. There were adventure dreams, too. Some dreams they liked and some were very scary.

I gave them a booklet to keep at their bedside that gave clues about how to remember dreams and a place where they could write some of their stories once they woke up. Here are the reminders included:

1. It helps to remember dreams if you go to bed when you are sleepy and get a good rest.
2. As you lie down, tell yourself that you will remember your dream when you wake up, and keep your paper with a pen near your bed to write them down or draw a picture of what you dream.
3. It also helps if you tell someone your dream soon after you wake up.

It seemed important for them to be excited about their trip, so I read stories about the adventures of other kids in their nighttime trips. My students really enjoyed hearing these stories and had lots of questions. This eased them into thinking about dreams as they looked at the pictures in the storybooks and saw how kids in the stories dealt with their dreams.

We wondered together, "Why do we dream?" Here are their answers:

1. To give us something to do while we sleep
2. To entertain us
3. To scare us

I suggested a few more:

4. To give us information
5. To teach us how to solve a problem.

So we began our journey into our nighttime adventures. Here are some of the dreams that the children told, and that we used for our exercises in class:

I was struck by lightning and I could see the lightning. It hit me on my forehead above my right eye. It felt like being shocked by an electric fence. I was very scared. Eight-year-old Amelia told this dream several times in class. She drew pictures of it and wanted to show the class where the lightning had shocked her, and frightened her.

Amelia also told this dream. *I dreamed I was a magic fluffy marshmallow jumping on clouds. I had a smiley marshmallow face and the sky was blue.* This was such a delightful dream. She wanted to draw it over and over again in different ways. She described the feeling of flying high in the clouds and how happy she was.

I was moving to a house. I was looking in a bedroom and I saw a zombie and then some zombies started chasing me and I woke up (Lotus, age 9). When asked her feelings, Lotus reported that she was scared and ran away.

I dreamed that Jurassic Park was real and the dinosaurs escaped and I saw the dinosaurs. When I woke up I was curious, excited, and scared (Tara, age 10).

Tara also reported, *There were ghosts in bottles of soap. I opened the bottles and was scared, then closed the bottles and threw them in the trash. When I woke up I felt a little scared, and also thought it was funny.*

In my dream my brother was taking something from me. I screamed, "no, don't take it, don't." It was a toy, and I talked in my sleep and got my toy back. When I woke up, I was glad. (Sonya, age 8). Sonya said she was embarrassed to show me her picture because her older brother had taken it away from her and written mean words and pictures all over the back.

I was in the forest and I was flying above all the trees and animals. Where I was flying I touched the treetops. It was cool (Autumn, age 10). Autumn drew a picture of herself flying saying, "Whee!" with the trees below. She named it "The Flight."

In my dream, I fell into a pit and yelled, then I woke up in the woods. I was scared. (Somaya, age 8).

Some Classroom Exercises with Dreams

Some of our journey included learning how to be creative with our imaginations, and since the children were learning, as a class, how to write stories, we used some of these ideas to help them write about their dreams. I asked them to use the following outline. A few of these stories became a vehicle for our dream drama:

1. Imagine your dream as a film and tell who the actors are.
2. Where does the dream take place?
3. What is unusual about this dream place?
4. Is the setting scary or calm or something else? Can you describe it?
5. What would you like to change in your dream story?
6. Why did you dream this? Is there a message for you?[8]

When writing, the kids would sit in small circles of six. They worked individually for a while and then asked for help from each other for words or ideas. They liked writing stories and especially getting and using ideas from their friends.

Many scary dreams came up on our journey. So as we sat together one evening around the campfire, we explored what happened in these dreams.

They shared what they did: "I run away"; "I scream and cry for help from my mom." "I turn and look at the zombie and say 'go away.'" I suggested that they could try something called "re-dreaming" or re-imagining. They could go back into a scary dream they have had and change the ending to one that makes them feel safe and in more control of the dream. Here is an example from author Jill Gregory: The students are allowed to dress like a dream character.

> One girl, Samantha, wore a long pointed hat. . . . She was portraying a large bluebird that bosses her and clings to her in her dreams two to three times a week. This had been going on for four years and the bird was becoming increasingly negative, to the point of attacking Samantha. . . . Samantha found ways to get that bird to sit and listen to her. She set some basic limits for the bird in terms of what she was willing to do for it, and gradually came to a place where she found another friend for the bluebird so it didn't come to her for all of its needs. In fact, she even imaged wings for the bird which the bird had told her was what he needed most. Although the bluebird was still a frequent symbol in her dreams, by the end of the course Samantha had a more positive relationship with it. Sometimes the bluebird would fly away and she would miss it.
>
> The wonderful thing about the approach of simply solving pictures and dream situations and helping our dream characters is that it works wonders for our lives without anyone needing to know who that bluebird represents in her real life and her dream life will improve without those correlations ever being drawn.[9]

In her book *Nightmare Help for Children from Children*, Ann Sayre Wiseman developed a technique using what she describes as a "paper stage" where the child draws the dream so that it can be seen visually by both the child and a guide:

1. The guide/helper can be a parent, teacher, or another who wishes to allow the child to safely re-dream this picture dream.
2. The guide talks first, if necessary, until the child feels safe enough.
3. The guide then asks questions to help the process.
4. Drawing the dream on paper usually creates a safe distance to begin the process.
5. It can sometimes help the dreamer to draw the guide into the picture for more safety, or to draw a shield, or become invisible. The dreamers often have their own ideas about this.
6. If the child feels confident and has permission, they often find their own solutions and resolution progressing beyond an unfinished sense of being stuck.

"Follow the dreamer's lead, stop at obstacles, respect fear and explore alternate routes and hang in there until the child finds a way out. . . . I have great faith in the sophistication and wisdom of children and their knowledge of what is right for them. Children have their own answers according to their own readiness if you will give them a chance to guide you"[10]

One morning on our journey, we went outside and enjoyed wandering. Since scary dreams were such a frequent occurrence for the children, I wanted to help them to remember that they have a safe place within themselves, even when things around them are frightening. So we sat in a large meadow, and I took them on a guided imagery journey to a safe and happy place, using words something like this:

Rub your hands together until they feel warm and then gently cover your eyes. Find a place where you can lie down and rest. See if you can imagine yourself in a place you love to go, maybe it is the ocean or maybe you go into a boat and sit in the middle of the water with a fishing pole. Maybe you like to walk in the woods near a lake where you can see the blue water. Feel the wind blowing around you and the sun shining. Are you by yourself or is there someone with you, a friend, a pet, or someone else you really like to be with? Just relax there sitting down under a tree or wherever you are. I'll give you a little time to just be there. Now come back to the meadow, where you can feel the ground under you, and the air around you, and sit up.

"Now get up and stretch. Then sit down again and take this paper. Write a description of this happy place. Describe a kind of dream you might like to have about this place. Remember that you can ask anytime at night for a dream about a safe and happy place." We then shared about our happy and safe places. One girl imagined herself up in the branches of a large tree among the birds. Another was lying down on a float in a pond looking up at the sky.

At the end of our session together, I reminded the children that there is a place in their imagination that they can go whenever they want to feel good, safe, and happy. I said to them: "Suppose you are unhappy with your friend, or someone was mean to you, or your parents have punished you for something you did wrong. Even when things are very hard or you feel scared, you can find inside yourself strength and peace."

The last days of our trip together were approaching. In spite of their restlessness as school was ending, these last two experiences become their favorites: dream drama and their superheroes selection. We have a sharing of dreams and then decide who would like to have their dream acted out. We select two dreams. I have brought in my suitcase for our journey with several scarves and masks and fabrics they can make into costumes. We start with a dream by Tanya, age nine. She wrote the following story:

Underwater at a Cottage

Once upon a time, I went to a pond with my friend, Tanya. We dove in and something grabbed us. We tried to get out but we could not. The thing pulled us farther down each time, and then we escaped and swam up to the surface. We were in a totally different place. We walked to a little cottage. Five werewolves attacked and captured us, and then we got away and ran back to the cottage. Then we went back to the pond and we dove back into the pond, and something grabbed us again and we got away and we swam back up the surface.

Tanya decided she wanted to be the main character in the dream. She assigned the different parts. Someone with a large, blue piece of fabric became the water. She decided who would be the narrator and where in the area the scenes would take place. The class was instructed that Tanya was in charge and would direct the action. The students got into their parts, and after the dream was enacted, we gathered to talk about it. I asked the dreamer if she learned anything that she did not know before acting the dream. She said, "I learned that it was much more fun to act out than to have the dream itself, and I could get away from the wolves and the things that grabbed at my legs with my friend."

The second dream was by Amelia, age eight.

"I lived in a very large fancy house with two circular staircases. There was a bedroom upstairs where my friend and I were sleeping. In the night, zombie arms came out of a cupboard on the wall and my friend and I got up and ran out of the room closing the door. A little boy (who in waking life attended the school in a lower grade and was mean to her and others) came over and I told him that the safest room was in the bedroom upstairs and I took him there and closed the door. Then all the zombies came out and scared him until he ran away."

The dreamer decided how her dream would be acted out and we proceeded. After the excitement of the drama, we settled down and gathered in a circle. I asked again what she knew now that she did not know before the drama. She responded, "I liked being mean to that little boy because he is such a bully and hurts us in the playground."

Acting out their dreams sparked many more dreams and they were excited about acting out more dreams. They did not want the journey to be over! What I loved is that they learned what they needed to know through the dramas, and their friends learned along with them. They all wanted to be the zombies, perhaps as a way of exploring their own fears related to having zombies or other monsters in their own dreams.

We had been reading stories about an imaginary figure that can come to help them in a scary dream to make them feel safer. On our last day as we were sitting looking out at a pond, I asked them who their "superhero" or dream protector might be. If they could call on a protector, who did they imagine it might be? Each one had a very unique figure. Here are some: two lions one on each side; the wind-spirit; a hippogriff; a dragon-unicorn; the family cat; an eagle; a black panther; a bear; and two pet dogs. Hearing these, I had an idea of what I might give them as we met for the final class. I had previously taken a picture of each one of them as if they were sleeping. Using their pictures, I made each one a card, which I presented to them on our way back to the classroom after our journey, telling them they might like to hang the card above their bed with their particular protector and a poem.

For example, I wrote this statement: "I am a powerful black panther and I am here to protect you from nightmare creatures. I am a guardian sent to you tonight. Do not be afraid in a dream. No one can bring you harm as I am your protector and guardian." I included a poem from *The Man in the Moon*, excerpted below:

> We will watch over the children of Earth [. . .]
> We will guard with our lives their hopes and dreams[11]

As we were saying goodbye to our nighttime adventure together, we did one final playful exercise using cards of dream characters made by dream expert and psychologist, Patricia Garfield, PhD. She had written a poem on the back of each card, and since the class loved to dress up, I asked them to choose a card and dress up like that figure while I read the poem. This allowed them to do something active and also to learn more about dreams and ideas about dreams. The girls and boys selected a picture to act out, and had fun imagining themselves in the roles. The students all now seemed eager to learn more, and wanted to act out more dreams and find ways to work with their own "scary" ones.

Some Ideas for Interacting with Children and Their Dreams

Here are a few more thoughts and ideas that might be useful for interacting with children and their dreams:

1. "Close bonds with parents often make it difficult for a child to tell whose feelings they are feeling. Empathy can be confusing: when parents are afraid for their children, not only does it add to the child's fears, it interferes with the child's ability to risk new things on their own."[12]

2. "If your child is scared to go to sleep, listen, reassure them and see what might help. If they fear the dark, try a flashlight and use it to make the dark fun with some kind of game; do a treasure hunt searching for things that glow in the dark; get a 'monster spray'; involve the child in coming up with ideas; discuss the fears in the daylight and set some limits as needed."[13]

3. "If something is YUCKY, take them outside and have them spit it out."[14]

4. Draw pictures of things your child loves, or cut them from magazines with their help. Fill a box with them, and have your child select a picture to think about while falling asleep.

5. It is important for parents and other adults to aid children by giving them a place to talk about their dreams as a real experience. One mother asks her children three questions each morning: Did you remember your dream? What was the dream about? Was the dream in color?[15]

6. Try having the child make a mask with a paper plate of a scary dream figure and act it out, then maybe burn it, or ask the child what he wants to do with it.

7. Settle children with soothing relaxation before bedtime. This may be the most important time a parent spends with their child. Provide them physical comfort; bless them with some ritual to guard them in the night. Give them a feeling of being very important and loved. Tuck them in![16]

Dreaming the Future

In this chapter, I introduced the idea of placing the dreams of our children in the context of the community in which they live and grow and interact with others. This includes family, friends, playmates, neighbors, birds, pets, movie images, and all the other myriad images seen in waking and dreaming life. Their imaginations are active and are constantly teaching them about our world, as we see in the dream story about the girl and her bird.

My dream in childhood of going to Africa created my lifelong desire to work with children and later to help them with their dreams. Working and playing with dreams can help children to grow a life that is rich and full of wisdom, adventure, and fun. Children love to use their imagination and to explore their dreams, especially through dream drama. This exploration can help them with their unique problems and it can help us all to see our own influence. Children see the world and all that is around them with new eyes. If we encourage them, we too can grow in new ways that not only make us more effective as parents but as people in the world.

For children, as for the rest of us, the weather sometimes gets rough and windy, sometimes very scary. We can help them to find safe spaces where they can work out the stresses and pressures, the traumatic life events that often cause them to have nightmares. As Patricia Garfield notes: "Nightmares are designed to wake you up. Drawing pictures and letting the dream speak gives you more power over the dream."[17]

Children have their own creativity and imagination that brings new solutions to problems. Their gifts are new. We can learn to honor their dreams, and them as individuals, as they create their own identity; an identity with which to better our world. If we could create a new generation of dreamers, what might they bring to this world so in need of new and creative ideas? If we assist children in gaining the deep insights dreams offer in understanding our emotions and our larger world, we could not offer them any more wondrous gift of love. What children dream holds hope for the future of this world.

Notes

1. Patricia Garfield, *Your Child's Dreams* (NY: Ballantine, 1984), 25–28.
2. Jonathan Gottschalk, *The Storytelling Animal* (New York: Houghton Mifflin, Harcourt, 2012), 84.
3. K. Ijams and L. D. Miller, "Perceptions of Dream Disclosure: An Exploratory Study," *Communications Studies* 51, 2000, 135–148.
4. Ibid.
5. Jill Gregory, "Bringing Dreams to Kids," *Dream Network Journal* 7(2), 1987, unpaginated.
6. Ibid.
7. www.Bluemountainschool.net\facts, 2015.
8. Brenda Mallon, *Dream Time with Children* (UK: Jessica Kingsley Publishers, 2002), 55.
9. Gregory, "Bringing Dreams to Kids."
10. Ann Sayre Wiseman, *Nightmare Help for Children by Children* (California: Ten Speed Press, 1989), 9–11.
11. Willian Joyce, *The Man in the Moon* (New York: Simon & Schuster, Atheneum Books for Young Readers, 2011), unpaginated.
12. Wiseman, *Nightmare Help for Children*, 22.
13. J. A. Owens, and J. A. Mindell, *Taking Charge of Your Child's Sleep; The All-in-One Resource for Solving Sleep Problems in Kids and Teens* (New York: Marlow and Co., 2010).
14. Robert Moss, "The first things to know about children's dreams," (www.Beliefnet\Dreamgates, 2015).
15. Dream Emporium.com, "Helping Children with Their Dreams."
16. Garfield, *Your Child's Dreams*, 352–353.
17. Ibid., 27.

Bibliography

Blue Mountain School: www.Bluemountainschool.net\facts, 2015.
Cosgrove, Stephen. *The Dream Tree*. New York: Penguin Putnam Books for Young Readers, 1974.

Garfield, Patricia. *Your Child's Dreams.* New York: Ballantine, 1984.

Garrison, Christian. *The Dream Eater.* New York: MacMillan, 1978.

Gottschalk, Jonathan. *The Storytelling Animal.* New York: Houghton Mifflin, Harcourt, 2012.

Gregory, Jill. "Bringing Dreams to Kids." *Dream Network Journal* 7, nos. 2 & 3 (1987).

"Helping Children with Their Dreams." www.dreamemporium.com.

Ijams, K and L. D. Miller. "Perceptions of Dream Disclosure: An Exploratory Study." *Communications Studies* 51, 2000.

Joyce, William. *The Man in the Moon.* New York: Simon & Schuster, Atheneum Books for Young Readers, 2011.

Mallon, Brenda. *Dream Time with Children.* London: Jessica Kingsley Publishers, 2002.

Moss, Robert. "The First Things to Know about Children's Dreams." www.Beliefnet .com/dreamgates.

Owens, Judith A. and J. A. Mindell. *Taking Charge of Your Child's Sleep: The All-in-One Resource for Solving Sleep Problems in Kids and Teens.* New York: Marlow, 2010.

Wahl, Jan. *Humphrey's Bear.* New York: Henry Holt and Co., 1987/2005.

Wiseman, Ann Sayre. *Nightmare Help for Children by Children.* Berkeley: Ten Speed Press, 1989.

PART THREE

Extreme Dreams

CHAPTER EIGHT

The Power of Dreamwork with Traumatized Adolescents

David Gordon and Dani Vedros

Then, the man looked me in the eyes and shot me through the heart. In the dream I died and I woke up with a horrible pain in my chest.

Sam, age 15

Most of us have had such disturbing dreams at some time in our lives. Typically, we find ourselves asking how they can be so vivid, feel so real and yet have the potential to help us when they seem so punitive. Yet many mental health professionals have found that dreams and even nightmares can be profound sources of healing both in and out of the therapeutic setting.[1]

In this chapter, we will show how working with dreams offers several key benefits uniquely suited to treating teens who have experienced the trauma of abandonment or emotional, physical or sexual abuse. These benefits—also equally helpful when working with nontraumatized teens—include an easing of tension related to hierarchy and authority within the therapy relationship; a consequent increased mutual empathy between therapist and client; and a shared language of metaphor that is directly relevant and rooted in the adolescent's personal life experience. Lastly, dream imagery offers the client—no matter how severely limited in life experience or verbally impaired—an embodied ground of direct experience that profoundly compensates for such deficits. Indeed, as you will see, dreams can also offer traumatized and emotionally neglected adolescents a first-time experience of safety and love not previously experienced in waking life.

To illustrate this, we will describe the healing nature of dreamwork with three traumatized adolescents who were participating in a community-based treatment program.[2] The program provided treatment to adolescent sexual offenders under the age of 21. These teens also had extensive histories of multiple traumas including early parental abandonment, economic deprivation, and exposure to community violence as well as physical, emotional, and/or sexual abuse. Many of the teens had been deemed treatment failures in other programs.

In this setting, dreamwork was an adjunctive approach provided within individual therapy by Dani Vedros, LCSW, coauthor of this chapter. Dani is a clinical social worker who initially served as clinical director in the program in which these teens were receiving treatment. Currently, she is in private practice in Norfolk, Virginia, with her husband and coauthor, David Gordon, PhD, a clinical psychologist. David developed a model of dreamwork—Mindful Dreaming—utilized by Dani in working with the adolescents in this chapter.[3]

It should be said from the outset that far too little has been explored or written illustrating the process of dreamwork with this population of adolescents. Indeed, we have found few case studies in the literature.[4] However, we would be remiss to not reference a wholly fascinating account of such work with incarcerated adult felons offered by Reverend Jeremy Taylor in his book *Where People Fly and Water Runs Uphill.*[5]

Mindful Dreaming: The Dream as a Source of Novel Healing Experience

The approach employed by Dani in the case studies throughout this chapter is one which combines traditional methods of dreamwork in addition to our own unique Mindful Dreaming perspective. By traditional dreamwork we are referring to the accepted practice of asking for the dreamer's associations to the dream imagery. We also refer to the point of view practiced by the famed Swiss analyst Carl Jung in which the dream is seen as a positive source of guidance and healing.[6] The Jungian perspective is that dreams speak not in disguised symbols, but in the universal language of metaphor; a language accessible to everyone. Moreover the Jungian view—and ours—is that dreams function to clarify our waking life conflicts, expand our awareness and point the way to new, healthier perspectives and behavior.

Here's a simple example of image as metaphor: I dream that "I am driving the car that I owned when I was graduating from high school and on my way to college." The car I drive in this dream serves as a metaphor for an experience I recall having while driving—an experience of growing confidence, excitement, and a newfound feeling of independence and autonomy.

In other words, behind or within every dream image is an experience our psyche calls us to reengage with and to embrace in a visceral way before asking: "Why am I being prompted to remember this way of being in the world at this moment in my life?" Perhaps, if I have been feeling pessimistic about the challenges I am facing, the dream may be suggesting that I am nevertheless on the verge of something very positive, similar to the time when I graduated high school. Consequently, my anxiety must be unfounded and blinding me to this change. Employing the language of metaphor, dreams compensate for our conscious point of view, for better or worse.[7]

However, the key concept in working with any dream is the dream "experience." Often people working with their own dreams or those of others stop short of the real gift of the dream, which is the novel and visceral experience it provides; instead, the focus remains centered on the "meaning" of the dream.

Dream images are laden with novel experiences as well as experiences we have forgotten or from which we have distanced ourselves, but our subsequent thoughts about the dream serve to make that experience abstract. For example, if a young adolescent dreams of riding a wild horse in the early morning air through a mountain pasture of wild flowers, she may look back on that dream and wonder about the meaning of a wild horse and what wild flowers symbolize. By the time she has finished "thinking" about those "symbols," and looking them up in a symbol dictionary, the dream would be reduced to something "quite interesting." Yet, what has been lost is the direct *experience* of the dream which was one of amazement, immersion in the beauty of nature, a sense of innocence, untamed energy, and the freshness of early morning air. This is a medicinal experience the dreamer's psyche wants her to consciously embrace right now in her waking life and which is within her potential to do.

Though thinking creates wonderful possibilities to ponder, our thoughts flatten and dry up the experience we contemplate. In fact, from the standpoint of the approach we call Mindful Dreaming, our nightly dreams teach us to stay mindful of the myriad thoughts that stand in the way of our own natural process of healing and growth, thoughts that limit our *experience* of what and who we are. Indeed, the characters who populate our dreams—whether human, animal, or spirit forms—are actually mentors helping us to become more conscious and mindful of the suffering our habits of thought create.

The notion that our thoughts are at the root of our suffering is the focus of a highly researched and effective psychological treatment known as cognitive therapy.[8] Mindful Dreaming takes this perspective a step further and demonstrates that there are actually five core habits of thought at the root of human suffering that appear in both waking life and dreams. These are thoughts about distraction, control, judgment, attachment, and impatience—universally human problems, but an even greater source of suffering for troubled adolescents. Each type of thought yields its own unique form of suffering.

Five Core Habits of Thought at the Root of Suffering

Distraction

Often quite striking when one observes adolescents is the degree to which they appear bored, restless, and irritable. Much like adults, adolescents rarely question their "monkey mind" life. As though they were trapeze artists, they live their days swinging from place to place and thought to thought. Like adults, they rationalize this constant movement—their love of distraction—as a search for fulfillment that cannot quite be named. "It's out there somewhere, I'm sure." As time goes on, the unique suffering from thoughts of distraction can lead to a life that feels increasingly boring, empty, and unsatisfying.

Control

As adolescents and adults, each day of our life we nurture thoughts and plans to control and struggle for what we want, to make things turn out our way, and influence others—forcefully or diplomatically—to achieve the goals we desire. This is the approach our culture sanctions. From the moment we awaken we rarely question the need to maintain our guard, expect criticism and plan our defenses in order to remain in control.

Teens in emotional turmoil generally make control their prime objective in the venues of family and community. The normal adolescent developmental task of claiming independence and autonomy can be subverted into a chronic, unending battle for control, for being as free as possible from the influence of parents and authority figures. Like adults, these teens often succumb to the unique quality of suffering created by overreliance on thoughts of control: feelings of intense frustration, powerlessness, and hopelessness.

Judgment

The intention to judge is ever-present when we interact with others, no matter whether friend or foe. We judge how people believe, speak, look, act, and laugh. Yet, as a class, adolescents are particularly self-judging, if not self-hating. The truth is that no matter how hurtful our secret judgments of others, they rarely hold a candle to the cruelty we—and especially troubled adolescents—reserve for ourselves.

The unique suffering that arises with self-judging thoughts is routinely manifested in feelings of unworthiness, depression, anxiety, and despair—and of course, self-destructive impulses.

Attachment

It is no coincidence that Buddhists view our thoughts of attachment as a primary source of suffering. Our thoughts about attachment to the fleeting attributes of money, property, status, role, and self-image are by definition filled with the unique suffering that stems from impermanence: insecurity, and fear of loss.

But again, adolescence severely exacerbates this type of suffering, as in fact it is a proverbial time of anxiety about loss. Even healthy adolescents must endure loss of self-esteem and self-image through frequent experiences of social rejection, loss of status with peers, loss of trust (earned or unearned) from parents, loss of romantic attachments and, ultimately, the loss of childhood itself for more troubled adolescents.

In adolescence one has little inclination or understanding of how to bear the pain of grief. Without the ability to grieve and release thoughts of attachment one cannot clear a space in life to move on and grow.

Impatience

In the first half of life especially, we nurture the thought that we will not find what we desire or be what we want soon enough. Failing to smell the roses, we spend our present moments impatiently thinking about how much better things will be—must be—sometime in the future and how we must hurry and get there. All the more true for adolescents who, by definition, are constantly impatient about achieving the freedoms they desire and the independence they crave. But then what is left of the present moment—the only moment in which we live? Sadly, we often fail to notice the loss of life's joys found only in the now.

Five Core Healing Values

Mindful Dreaming teaches that our nightly dreams also offer us five healing values that are alternatives to our favorite habits of thought. To release distraction, our dreams prompt us to embrace stillness and self-reflection.

In place of our insistence upon control, we are called to surrender ego and allow ourselves to be led; to release judgment we must find compassion for our own suffering, not just that of others. Realizing the futility of attachment in an impermanent world, we must embrace grief and accept the sadness of loss, so that we can clear a space for new growth. Finally, we are rewarded for releasing impatience by embracing the gifts of the present moment, free of anxiety, and fear about what the future holds.

Mentors, whether human, animal, spirit forms, or nature herself, appear in our dreams encouraging us to embrace these five healing values. Indeed, our mentors are the embodiments of the change our psyche calls us to embrace. They challenge the ways we think because our five core habits of thought always underlie our suffering, blocking our growth, and healing.

Whether we respond with receptivity and openness to the call for a change in our thinking or with suspicion and resistance determines whether we experience our dream mentors as supportive and kind or as nightmare figures filling us with anxiety and dread. For this reason, even nightmares are not "bad" dreams, but rather dreams prompting necessary change toward which we feel resistant and frightened. The more resistant we feel the more threatening our mentors appear. The more receptive and open to the guidance of our mentors and the change they represent, the more they appear benevolent and wise. We will see examples of this in the following case studies.

Dreamwork with Three Traumatized Adolescent Clients

In the case studies you are about to read, we guide you through a brief summary of each adolescent's traumatic history and the dreams they shared in therapy. All identifying details have been changed to protect identity. We point out a few of the various forms dream mentors took, and the teens' attitudes toward their mentors. We will also look at the particular thoughts that sustained their suffering and the healing values that their dreams prompted them to embrace.

Before proceeding, it is important to note that the vast majority of children and adolescents who sexually offend do not go on to be pedophiles or adult offenders. Rather, they are young people with a multitude of severe emotional and psychosocial issues.

Frank

Frank had been born into a large family. He was the third oldest of five children. His mother was mildly mentally disabled, drug addicted, and depressed. His father left when Frank was 10 years old. All of the children were placed with foster families and, in the end, all but Frank had found a permanent home.

By the time Frank was 12 years old he had been placed in and rejected by multiple foster homes. He was hostile and depressed and had been diagnosed with a learning disability and ADHD. Now Frank was entering puberty, and in addition to other acting out behaviors, he began flashing his penis at male foster siblings. Eventually, he was placed in a residential program for juvenile sexual offenders.

When Frank entered our program, he was staying in an independent living group home. He was approaching his 18th birthday and was therefore mandated to leave the foster care system. Unsurprisingly, it was extremely difficult for him to express himself in therapy. However, we found that his dreams were especially beneficial in assisting him to transcend his overwhelming emotional and communication difficulties, while providing a novel ground of direct experience upon which to draw and envision a new life.

Frank's First Dream

Some of the people that work with me at McDonald's invited me to eat lunch at Hardee's. We ate together.

Understandably, Frank had been feeling that he would always be alone and could not imagine a future where he could create relationships and a support system that would approximate the feeling of family.

Yet, when asked which people from McDonald's were with him at Hardees in his dream, Frank brightened and indicated that they were the coworkers and a supervisor with whom he worked there and liked. And, when asked about his associations to Hardees, he identified it as a place "where they serve chicken, and chicken is what families eat together on Sunday afternoons."

Prompted to close his eyes, reenter his dream, and more fully experience the meal at Hardees, Frank experienced himself—thanks to his dream mentors—as sharing a family dinner at the table with coworkers. The feeling of connection and belonging to family now became tangibly and viscerally alive for him. He felt for the first time in his conscious memory the fulfillment and warmth of being accepted and cared for as families do. This was an epiphany for Frank whose thoughts about others were that they were always judging him unworthy—as he indeed judged himself. Yet, the dream experience was one of nonjudgment, in which he felt himself for the first time receiving compassion and acceptance. This is the gift of every dream: that some dysfunctional thought—in this case the thought of being judged—is either challenged or transcended and a corresponding healing experience, compassion, provided in its stead.

What Frank longed for was no longer an abstract idea proposed by an authority he could not relate to or fully trust. Rather the dream experience was a reality, sourced from within, and one that Frank could begin to embrace and feel capable of manifesting in his life.

Frank's Second Dream

Frank shared this next dream while feeling intense ambivalence about leaving his group home, a requirement mandated by his pending 18th birthday. He was now earning enough money at McDonald's to live independently, but he continued to act out in minor ways that delayed his departure. He denied that his behavior reflected any fear about leaving. Yet his unacknowledged judgmental thoughts about himself as inadequate to succeed, and this consequent self-sabotage of his own independence, went on for about four months. Then he brought the following dream to therapy:

> I was at the home and I noticed that some of the kids were missing parts of their bodies. I thought that they had lost them in violent ways. Other people in the group home were very angry. I thought: "I don't belong here."
> Then the police showed up and started chasing me. I was terrified and ran into the woods, but the cops chased me deeper and deeper. I found a ditch and tried to lay in it and go to sleep, but the cops kept driving by so I had to stay alert.

When helped to reenter the dream, Frank saw that he could easily identify with the residents in the group home who, like himself, felt angry and broken by the physical and emotional violence they had endured in their life. However, the support Frank was receiving in therapy and the renewed hope engendered by his dream of "eating at Hardees" helped him begin to move beyond the judgmental view of himself as defective and still in need of the structure and sanctuary of the group home setting. Now, contemplating his own words in the dream—"I don't belong here"—as his own and not the words of an authority figure or therapist encouraged Frank to accept the change he needed to embrace.

In Mindful Dreaming, it is an axiom that as our thoughts arise they create the unfolding reality in our dream and each new scene. Thus when Frank thought "I don't belong here," his dream mentors in the form of the seemingly hostile police appear suddenly and "chase" him away from his security and dependence on the group home. Ironically, the function of the police in waking life is to ensure an orderly and safe society: just what Frank needs to feel about the world he is moving toward. But he must be chased away because he judges himself inadequate to the new task of independence and still fears change. It is this fear of change that leads him to perceive his mentors as threatening, when in fact they are prompting him to leave the unhealthy place to which he is clinging. Frank's dream is urging him to release self-judgment and to find more compassion for himself by nurturing his own autonomy and independence.

Just as in fairy tales and fables, when the proverbial fool on his journey for the grail must "enter the wood in its darkest place," so too Frank finds himself in a new phase of his life, lost and frightened "in the woods." He rightly fears "falling asleep," as in dreams to fall asleep is often a metaphor for falling back into an unconscious state and avoiding change. His mentors, the police, assist him in this goal by constantly "driving by" and keeping him awake. Indeed, Frank must remain "alert" and vigilant in his quest to find his competence in the world.

This dream became the jumping off point and ongoing focus of discussion in therapy as Frank created a foundation for his future life. He was now able and highly motivated to discuss his fear of the "dark woods" of his future as an adult entering into the unknown without the external structure and rules he had lived with for so many years.

The last dream that Frank shared was toward the end of therapy. Remarkably, he was by now residing in an independent-living apartment and had been working at the same job for a year. He was planning to take job training classes at a local community college and he had his first girlfriend. He was 19 years old.

Frank's Third Dream

I was Spiderman swinging from building to building with my web. I shot my web but nothing came out. I fell to the ground. I was surprised that I didn't die! I was OK! I was really happy.

In this dream, Frank has become his own mentor. That is, he relies on his own resources to function in the world without assistance. This is not to say that he no longer needs the support and guidance of others, but that he has stabilized for the present moment at a very fulfilling level of competence, autonomy, and inner authority about his ability to function in society.

However, the dream narrative suggests that he has been holding the comforting view of himself as having somehow been graced with magical power. That is in fact the nature of the actual Spiderman story: a story about great though unearned power. Nevertheless, Frank's dream shows him a more potent truth. Upon losing his magical skills, he finds himself "back to earth." Often, falling down, falling back to earth, in a dream is metaphorically a call to release one's fears of everyday life and to become more grounded in one's own realistic strengths and weaknesses.

In waking life, having earned his way back into society, Frank in his dream is now surprised and overjoyed that he can stand on his own two feet so to speak. As a result, being in the world no longer feels like a mortal threat: "I didn't die!" This indeed is a cause for celebration and reason to be "really happy."

His final therapy sessions could now focus on the dream's assertion that his newfound abilities in life were not Spiderman magic or wishful thinking, but rather very real, down-to-earth skills on which he could truly rely.

Though Frank reported only three dreams, they provided a very frequent and ongoing reference for discussion about deserving compassion; not judgment. In this regard, the work of integrating a dream experience in waking life is always as important as the initial epiphany it offers.

It is worth reiterating that Frank's dreams were not "interpreted" and intellectually analyzed for him. Rather, he was prompted to feel into the guiding experiences they provided.

Sam

Sam had been removed from his mother's home during prepubescence because she was living with a convicted pedophile and it was suspected that Sam had been abused by this man. He was constantly removed from foster homes due to sexual acting out. At other times, he was returned to live with his mother, only to be removed again due to her continued abuse and neglect. As Sam fully entered puberty he became aggressive and intimidating toward others.

Sam was 15 years old and living in a foster home when he entered our treatment program. He had been in the foster care system many years and had been with at least eight different therapists. Discharge reports always included a negative prognosis. Sam portrayed himself as cold and uncaring and would brag about his risk-taking and indifference to consequences. He was oppositional and defiant in the extreme.

After a few months of weekly meetings, Sam shared his first and only dream—a dream that had remained with him since early childhood.

Sam's Dream

I always remember this dream from when I was around six or seven. Me and some friends were playing video games in the living room. We all heard a noise from my mom's bedroom. Some of the kids went to the door to find out what the noise was. Then a dark man jumped out and started shooting everyone. The other kids fell to the ground and they all died. Then, the man looked me in the eyes and shot me through the heart. In the dream I died and I woke up with a horrible pain in my chest.

To assess the nature of the dysfunctional habit of thought being addressed by a dream one need only look at the mood at the end of the dream, as our thoughts create our mood.

In the previous case, Frank's dream of being chased by cops had ended in a fearful mood typical of judgment dreams because in such dreams we project our own critical thoughts and judgments on to our mentors, and then fear them.

However, Sam's dream ends with an experience of sadness and loss. A sad mood at the end of a dream suggests that it is an attachment dream. Attachment dreams point to our attachment to an object, idea, relationship, or psychological defense that needs to be released for our own continued growth. In this dream, Sam is being prompted to release attachment to the defense of denial about a painful loss so that healthy grieving and healing can occur.

Sam's dream explains in visual terms how he was hurt with a shot to the heart—meaning metaphorically that his heart had been broken. With this broken heart, his openness to love and being loved had closed down by the time of the dream when he was six or seven years of age. It is reasonable, given the known history, to speculate as well that the dark man responsible for this was the pedophile with whom Sam lived. Yet, the man also serves as a mentor who provides the impetus to resolve a lifelong trauma through reenactment in the dream of the emotional wound that needs healing—a shot to the heart—as opposed to the literal sexual violation.

By being helped to gently reenter the dream experience of his own murder, Sam was enabled to feel much needed compassion for himself, break through his bravado, and acknowledge that he had been severely hurt. For the first time in his life he began to address his history of trauma and abuse and embrace his vulnerability, sadness, and loss.

Thomas

Thomas had been released from a juvenile correctional facility on his 18th birthday and was mandated by the court to participate in therapy. He had been placed in the facility at age 12, following a conviction for sexual assault. He had not successfully completed the sex offender program in Corrections and had committed multiple violent offenses while detained.

He was being released because the facility could not hold him beyond age 18. None of the local step-down facilities would take him because of his reputation.

When it became clear that Thomas was going to be released into the community regardless of whether a treatment program would accept him, he was allowed into our program. Sincere participation in the program was not a requirement of probation, so Thomas knew that just as he had waited out the system in Corrections, he could easily wait out his six month probation in the program. Surprisingly, after a month of unproductive meetings, he agreed to share a dream at Dani's request.

Thomas's Dream

At the time I had this dream I was thirteen. I was lying in the time-out room in my underwear. The floor was hard cement. I had never been so cold in my life. I had been fighting and acting crazy. I was so pissed off at being there I wanted to die and I was planning to fight until I was killed or killed someone else.

I fell asleep on that floor and in my dream God came to me and he stroked my head and it felt really warm. I realized I was going to be OK, and that I was going to make it out of there. I kinda felt loved for the first time. He didn't say a word to me, it was just the touch.

I woke up crying. I wanted to live and to get out. I knew I was supposed to do something with my life but I didn't know how or what I could do.

This simple, clear dream was emotionally and spiritually transformative. The dream had provided this young man with a direct experience of hope, redemption, and inherent sacredness as an individual at a very critical point in his life. Its healing power had lain dormant however, until he was afforded the opportunity to process the dream's wisdom with Dani.

With the dream as the ultimate authority, tensions around power and hierarchy were no longer relevant. Thomas could relax and trust his therapist to provide the help his dream told him he deserved. His dream also provided a grounding and centering experience to which he could return whenever he was feeling difficult emotions, by simply reentering the dream in his memory.

For the first time in his life, Thomas was able to express and fully experience his fear, anxiety, grief, shame, deep sadness, and loss. Through this process, he changed a lifelong pattern of acting out aggression and hostility.

Within the Mindful Dreaming paradigm, one can see that Thomas's dream helped him to release his tight grip on control, embrace humility, and follow guidance. This single dream prompted him to release judgment of himself and others and to find greater self-caring and compassion.

He released attachment to his old identity as an enraged, but powerless victim of others, and began to accept his losses, embracing and honoring his long-held grief. Finally, the dream facilitated this profound transformation by directing Thomas's attention to a still, quiet place within, away from the distractions of his life, to focus more productively and patiently on the work of therapy.

Thomas remained in treatment for an additional 10 months. When he ended therapy, he was less stuck in the past and more actively engaged now in his present life: working full time, taking community college classes at night, and looking for an apartment.

* * *

In these three cases the use of dreamwork allowed traumatized, angry adolescent boys with no apparent history or capacity for self-reflection, and no motivation or interest in treatment to make relatively rapid and positive changes in therapy.

Sadly, oppositional and defiant adolescents are often approached with judgment and fear even by the professionals who intend to provide healing. Dreamwork ameliorates this mutual impasse, as the therapist and client recognize the dream as the authority in the therapeutic work and the dream belongs to the client. Dreamwork also provides a shared language of metaphor to be used by the client and therapist that is directly relevant to the client's experience.

Most profoundly, dreamwork provides a ground of direct healing experience that words alone cannot convey, let alone create. The powerful therapeutic effect of these dreams was especially moving given the significant verbal impairment and history of severe abuse suffered by these young men. In the case of Frank and Thomas, the experience of safety and love occurred for the first time in their lives in their dreams. In Sam's case, the dream opened him up to feeling love after a trauma early in life had closed him down. His grief became accessible to therapeutic exploration.

We can see that using these techniques with traumatized adolescent offenders served to create a therapeutic space rich with compassion that facilitated trust and created the potential for deep and lasting healing. Their dreams and the act of sharing them opened these boys for the first time in their life to the experience of trust, hope, healing, and growth.

Dream Sharing with Emotionally Healthy Adolescents

The techniques employed in this chapter can also be used by parents who wish to enhance communication, form a deeper bond with their teens, and help them find an inner source of guidance and support. Here are a few basic steps that can be followed at home, but you can also read about this subject in greater depth in the existing literature.[9]

- Help your teen explore the metaphorical meaning of the dream images. You might begin by pointing out that we speak in metaphor every day. For example, we may say that someone "missed the bus" when they refused to take an opportunity given to them. Or, we say that "I'll cross that bridge when I come to it" as a reference to a time of transition in life. These metaphors have the same meaning when they appear in a dream as "A bus I just missed" or "A bridge I crossed."
- Then you may want to ask: "Is there anything familiar about that experience?" or "Is there anywhere in your waking life where you've missed an opportunity or feel you are transitioning or changing?
- Rather than interpreting or telling your teen what you think the dream means, prompt your teen to talk about and feel into the images and experiences that arose in the dream. In general, it is best to ask questions such as, "You said that you were on a train in your dream. What is that experience like for you? What is the best and worst part of being on a train?"
- Remember that every dream figure is a mentor offering healthy change. If the dream character is perceived as frightening or alien in any way you may want to ask, "In moderation, what would be the good part if you felt a very tiny bit like that character in your dream? For example, a dream of being chased by a psychopath may lead to a question about what might be good in moderation about being a psychopath. The answer for example, may be, "Well I wouldn't always be feeling so guilty about everything."

In sum, dreamwork is a powerful source of guidance and healing. We believe that it should be considered ideal when working with adolescents, in that the process transcends the typical pitfalls inherent in working with this population. Most profoundly, the method of reentering and embodying the dream experience minimizes the challenge of persuading the adolescent that life can be experienced in a new way. Rather, the embodying of dream imagery is largely sufficient to transcend our conditioned thoughts and to reengage more wholeheartedly with life. It was the famed author Henry Miller who wrote, "The moment one gives close attention to anything, even a blade of grass, it becomes a mysterious, awesome, indescribably magnificent world in itself."

This is the opportunity our nightly dreams offer us all.

Notes

1. Deirdre Barrett, *Trauma and Dreams* (Cambridge, MA: Harvard University Press, 2001); Kelly Bulkeley, *Dreams of Healing: Transforming Nightmares into Visions*

of Hope (Mahwah, NJ: Paulist Press, 2003); Earnest Hartmann, *Dreams and Nightmares: The Origin and Meaning of Dreams* (New York: Perseus Publishing, 2000).

2. John A. Hunter, Stephen A. Gilbertson, Dani Vedros, Michael Morton, "Strengthening Community-Based Programming for Juvenile Sexual Offenders: Key Concepts and Paradigm Shifts," *Child Maltreatment* 9, no. 2 (2004): 177–189.

3. David Gordon, *Mindful Dreaming: A Practical Guide for Emotional Healing through Transformative Mythic Journeys* (Wayne, NJ: Career Press, 2006).

4. Gordon Halliday, "Dreamwork and Nightmares with Incarcerated Juvenile Felons," *Dreaming: Journal of the Association for the Study of Dreams* 14, no. 1 (2004): 30–42.

5. Jeremy Taylor, *Where People Fly and Water Runs Uphill: Using Dreams to Tap the Wisdom of the Unconscious* (New York: Grand Central Publishing, 1993).

6. C. G. Jung, *Dreams* (Princeton, NJ: Princeton University Press, 1974).

7. Ibid.

8. Judith S. Beck, *Cognitive Behavior Therapy, Second Edition: Basics and Beyond* (New York: The Guilford Press, 2011).

9. Alan Siegel and Kelly Bulkeley, *Dreamcatching: Every Parent's Guide to Exploring and Understanding Children's Dreams and Nightmares* (New York: Three Rivers Press,1998); Kelly Bulkeley and Patricia M. Bulkley, *Children's Dreams: Understanding the Most Memorable Dreams and Nightmares of Childhood* (Lanham, MD: Rowman & Littlefield Publishers, 2012).

Bibliography

Barrett, Deirdre, Ed. *Trauma and Dreams.* Boston: Harvard University Press, 2001.

Bulkeley, Kelly. *Dreams of Healing: Transforming Nightmares into Visions of Hope.* Mahwah, NJ: Paulist Press, 2000.

Hartmann, Earnest. *Dreams and Nightmares: The Origin and Meaning of Dreams.* New York: Perseus Books, 2000.

Jung, C. G. *Dreams.* Princeton, NJ: Princeton University Press, 1974.

Jung, C. G. *Memories, Dreams, Reflections.* New York: Vintage Books, 1989 Reissue Edition.

Jung, C. G. *The Meaning and Significance of Dreams.* Sigo Press. https://openlibrary.org/subjects/person:c._g._jung_(1875–1961).

Siegel, Alan and Kelly Bulkeley. *Dreamcatching: Every Parent's Guide to Exploring and Understanding Children's Dreams and Nightmares.* New York: Three Rivers Press, 1998.

Siegel, Alan. *Dreams That Can Change Your Life: Navigating Life's Passages through Turning Point Dreams.* New York: Berkley Books, 1992.

Taylor, Jeremy. *Where People Fly and Water Runs Uphill: Using Dreams to Tap the Wisdom of the Unconscious.* New York: Grand Central Publishing, 1993.

CHAPTER NINE

Dreams of Bereaved and Grieving Children: The Impact of Death on Dreams

Brenda Mallon

There was a knock on the door. I answered it and it was my dad. He looked really well and he had a suitcase. He said, "I've just come to say I'm OK and I'm going off on holiday now. I just wanted you to know I'm all right.

Billy's dream of his dead father

I began working with bereaved children over 30 years ago when I first trained as a counselor. My passionate interest in dreams and the study of their therapeutic value led me to use them as part of the healing process when working with both adults and children. I have been privileged to learn so much from the thousands of people who have helped in my work and research that has culminated in my most recent book, *Working with Bereaved Children and Young People.*[1]

In this chapter I hope to show how we can help children who dream about death and the deceased, and those who may struggle with distressing dreams. It includes practical strategies that anyone who cares for children can use. Each response to death is unique and we can see how trauma, sudden death and suicide affect children and their dreams. I also hope you can share the journey with children who have experiences of visitation dreams where the deceased loved one brings healing connection. As always, the most important aspect of dreamwork and dreamplay is to listen to the children and respond to their needs.

I have found that children are often fascinated by dreams. As they grow and develop, their understanding of dreams changes. Many young children think that dreams come from outside themselves; as four-year-old Eve told me, "They are pictures in my pillow." She believed that, as she slept, pictures rose from her pillow and filled her head with monsters and magic.[2] Later, children become more aware that dreams are part of each person, as 12-year-old Lucy describes: "Dreams tell us what we are really like inside. Our subconscious is letting us know what we think."[3] They learn that dreams are linked to their own experiences. As noted researcher Worden states, "Children who maintained a connection with the (deceased) parent through dreams and feeling watched knew, for the most part, that these experiences were coming from somewhere inside themselves."[4]

When a child has been bereaved, his or her dreams may reflect the impact of this major event. If we care for children, we must also care about their dreams and help them to harness their healing power.

We live in an "Assumptive World."[5] We assume that our routine and daily life will carry on as it has always done. However, that world can be shattered at any moment, as traumatic events demonstrate. Children assume they will live with their family, go to school, and see their friends. Yet when a traumatic event happens, particularly if it results in the death of a parent, caregiver, or sibling, their world is irrevocably changed and will never be the same again. Their security is shattered; their world is turned upside down. The transition they make after a death is the "work" of mourning; children and young people look to adults to move through a territory that has no map and they have to learn to make meaning of it.[6]

The poet Edna St. Vincent Millay's verse from 1915[7] expresses how her waking loss found its way into her sleeping consciousness:

> Where you used to be, there is a
> hole in the world,
> Which I find myself walking around in the daytime,
> And falling into at night.

Dreams relating to bereavement may occur before death as a form of anticipatory grief and children who are living with a terminally ill member of their family may have dreams that are distressing. They may be fearful about what will happen after the death. It is important to support the child by talking about their fears, offering whatever reassurance that can be given and helping them to communicate their feelings to those around them. Silence and lack of inclusion isolate the child and hinder resilience.

Dreams may also come immediately after the death of a loved one as a reaction to the loss, and dreams of the deceased may occur for the rest of the child's lifetime reflecting the nature of their relationship with the deceased.[8] Dreaming of the deceased has been shown to facilitate the grieving process.[9] I have found that children who are grieving recall their dreams more readily than those who are not, a view supported by other research.[10] Grieving is not a linear process and bereaved children will revisit the death and the narrative of what happened at different points in their life.

Continuing Bonds

> Come to me in my dreams, and then
> By day I shall be well again!
> For then the night will more than pay
> The hopeless longing of the day.
>   Matthew Arnold, 1855.[11]

Dreams may reveal the continuing bonds that connect the child to the person who has died. They also show that grieving does not have a finite time limit. In fact, "the dead are a positive resource to be drawn on by the living."[12]

Mel was eight when she told me of her dreams:

I used to dream of my cousin who was four years old when she died. She was very close to me. After her death I dreamt that she woke me up and we used to play with her dolls. I was always sad after that dream. I wanted to die so I could live with her and play with her. I always played with her in my dreams, for a year after she died. Now, I still occasionally have dreams of walking up stairs and meeting her. Sometimes, I still wish I could live with her.

Phyllis Silverman and her colleagues carried out seminal research into children's experience of bereavement.[13] One aspect of the grieving process is the establishment of a set of memories, feelings, and actions referred to as "constructing the deceased." They identified five stages that reflected the child's efforts to maintain the connection to the deceased parent:

- First was locating the deceased, usually "in heaven": "I know Granddad's happy in heaven with Granny, but I just wish he was here with us too." Paul, age nine.[14]
- Second, experiencing the deceased, for instance believing the deceased is watching them: "I sometimes smell her perfume and feel that she is with me." Gwen, 18, whose mother died a year before.

- Third, reaching out to the deceased in thoughts: "I'll see her. Sometimes at night, I talk to her when I say my prayers, and I cry, she tells me not to cry and that maybe someday I'll see her."[15]
- Fourth, waking memories; Sam's father died in a tragic accident when Sam was aged seven. When I asked him if he had any special memories he said, "Yes, my Dad taught me how to whistle. Do you want me to whistle for you?" That memory and that skill will be part of Sam for all his life and I will never forget hearing that little boy whistle.
- Fifth, cherishing linking objects. "I've got my Mum's photographs and a CD she liked. I keep them in my Memory Box and look at them when I'm missing her." Carl, 14.

These continuing bonds provide an emotional anchor for the young person as they sail in the stormy seas of bereavement.

In working with bereaved children we can help foster these connections, these continuing bonds. "Bereavement," Silverman and her fellow researchers conclude, "should not be viewed as a psychological state that ends or from which one recovers; rather, it should be understood as a cognitive and emotional process that occurs in a social context of which the deceased is part."[16] This is the reason why it is important not to use the term *closure* in relation to bereavement because the continuing bonds may never be broken nor cease. They will always be part of the child's story and part of his or her history.

Themes in Children's Dreams

Most children experience nightmares between the ages of three and sixteen. The usual themes are fear of separation, fear of being abandoned, being injured, or attacked. Also, "shape-shifting" dreams, in which a familiar person transforms into a frightening person or animal, are not uncommon.[17] For example, 10-year-old Paul told me, "I dream that men and women change into monsters and eat other people. They eat heads and arms and legs. I hate these bad dreams."

Julie had the following nightmare when she was seven years old. It includes shape-shifting and a feeling of horror followed by the dismay of not being believed:

> The dream took place in my Nana's house. I walked into the large bedroom where my Nana sleeps and found my Dad standing beside the bed dressed in trousers, shirt and tie, but he had a monster's head. His hair was on end, he had a greeny-gray disfigured face and he had large fangs dripping saliva. I was petrified. I just stood there shocked that my loving, caring Dad had changed into an evil

*monster. I ran screaming into the living room where my mum was and I told her
what I saw. She laughed when we went back into the bedroom because my Dad
was back to normal. When my mum started to laugh at me, for thinking my
Dad was a monster, I cried even more. I was annoyed because I really did see
him and I was hurt because no one believed me.*

These dreams reveal the growing awareness of duality of human beings. We
are complex creatures who can be heroic or demonic and such dreams
reflect that complexity. Part of growing up is to recognize that those we love
may have negative aspects as well as positive sides, which applies to all
human beings.

Deep fear, which surfaces in some dreams, may not be the literal details of
the death but may be expressed symbolically. For example, the dreamer may
be overwhelmed by a flood or tidal wave, be attacked by people or wild animals, be caught in a fire with no way of escape, be in a plane which is about
to crash or be caught in a hurricane. The underlying sense in the dream is that
events are beyond the control of the dreamer, just as the death was.

Overwhelmed by Trauma

Trauma occurs when a sudden, unexpected or completely extraordinary
event overwhelms the child's ability to cope and creates feelings he cannot
control. Trauma is different from everyday stress in a child's life because it
comes out of the blue and the child has no time to prepare for it. Frequently
feelings of helplessness swamp the child and there do not seem to be any
obvious ways that the child can make a difference. Such feelings of powerlessness undermine the child and these feelings find their way into the
dreams and nightmares of traumatized children.

Traumatic bereavement may induce recurring nightmares and fear of
sleep. By enabling the child to gain mastery of their dream material, in
exploration, drawing, creative writing or storytelling, we can show how
dreams can be part of a healing process. An example from my own practice
shows how you can use these techniques.

Jessie's 12-year-old brother Emile, was killed by the driver of a van as he
tried to cross the road following their older brother Timothy. Timothy wit-
nessed the accident and the death of his brother and was traumatized by the
experience. While Jessie did not witness the accident she felt the intense
grief of her parents and brother. Her mother brought her to see me when
Jessie was having trouble sleeping.

Jessie, aged six, said she did not like to go to sleep because she had sad
and frightening dreams. She told me, "I dreamt a lion came into my

bedroom and ate Emile. I couldn't stop the lion." She looked very unhappy, on the verge of tears. I asked her to draw her dream. She drew a large lion with her brother in its mouth. When I asked her if she would like to change the dream she said that she would like to change it so that Emile killed the lion and saved his own life. She drew a fresh picture of a smiling brother holding a smiling tiger with herself shouting out in joy. The tiger was reduced in size while her brother looked strong. She was pleased with the change and told me that she missed her brother very much. There was no need to go further in this dreamwork because she had found her own way to resolve the pain of the dream.

I saw Jessie a couple more times. In the next session she drew a picture of herself dancing with her brother in her dream. Both were smiling and Jessie clearly enjoyed her renewed contact with her brother. Jessie had no further problems sleeping because, though she knew her brother was dead, she knew she could talk about him and the memories she has of him and that, if she had frightening dreams, she could draw a happier ending. In working with dreams in bereavement we can give children tools to empower and enrich them.

The Impact of Suicide and Sudden Death

The impact of death by suicide may profoundly affect children and young people, often leaving them with emotional trauma as well as feelings of guilt, anger, shame, and confusion. Donna Schuurman, when executive director of the Dougy Center in the United States of America, recounted the words of Philip, a teenager with whom she was working. Philip described a meeting he had had with his deceased mother in a dream. In the dream he asked her why she had killed herself. She told him that she knew she would never be well, and that she wanted him to have a life free of her antics and unpredictable behavior. Philip said, "So, I told her I understood and forgave her."[18] Such dreams bring the opportunity for reconciliation and renewal.

Helena was 10 when her father died by suicide. She said: "I was so tired when I first knew. I was scared to do anything at first—going out, going back to school. When I went back, they asked me how my Dad died. At first I didn't tell them, then when I got used to it, I told them." Thoughts about suicide and sudden death may be unspeakable, the child literally cannot speak of what has happened, as Helena's experience shows. If this is the case, these feelings will be voiced in some other way and for children it is often in dreams that the unspeakable asserts its voice. To assist at this point we need to help children gain emotional mastery. In dreams, this may be to fully explore the imagery, to find different endings, draw healing outcomes—to bring the fears from the dark night of the dream into the light of day where the child can be supported to explore them.

I saw Alice, aged seven, when I was a bereavement counselor at the Grief Centre in Manchester. She told me that she was with her mother, her younger sister, and other members of her family going to school when her sister was killed. It was like every other school day morning but her world changed. She said her little sister let go of her mother's hand and was hit by a silver car. Since that time, Alice has had recurring dreams of a silver car hitting and killing her sister. She blamed herself. She believed she could have done something to save her sister's life. Alice drew pictures of her dreams for me and we looked at where everyone was when the car struck. It became clear to Alice that she was furthest away and could not have done anything to prevent the death. We talked about this over many sessions and gradually her feelings of guilt reduced, although she was sad and still missed her sister. She also felt ashamed that after the accident, she started to wet the bed again as she had done as a younger child. When I explained that children often go back to earlier behavior after such a traumatic event and that it was not her fault, she felt more positive and the bedwetting stopped.

David's brother was killed in a cycling collision. After this happened David had recurring dreams in which death was the repeated theme. The most frightening one, he told me, was one in which all his family were killed in a car crash and he was the only survivor. "Only I lived and I was paralyzed so I couldn't kill myself." The traumatic death of his brother left David feeling completely powerless, symbolized by his paralysis. His fears that other deaths would happen is not unusual: many children and young people believe that once someone has died, other deaths will follow. As one bereaved child asked me, "Is it my turn next?" Listening to such fears and addressing them are all part of the process of renewal as the child makes sense of life and death.

Fear and Anxiety in Dreams

I used to see my mum dying in my sleep and I would not go to school the next day because I was scared

Emma, 14

Emma's dream came after her parents divorced and she had to live with her father and his new wife. In her waking life she wants to be with her mother and her dreams reflect her fear that something will happen to her mother and Emma will be isolated and bereft. The fact that she does not want to go school after this dream alerts us to anxiety that can be triggered by dreams. Dream feelings spill over into waking life which is why it is a good idea to regularly ask children about how they slept and to ask about their dreams. This provides an opportunity for them to communicate their feelings and anxieties.

Visitation Dreams

> So, if I dream I have you, I have you.
>
> John Donne. Elegy 10, "The Dream."[19]

Visitation dreams are those dreams in which the deceased "visit." They often have an intensity that other dreams do not share—a kind of hyperreality. When death has happened, the child may dream of the deceased returning and this can be a comfort or a curse; the child may believe that the dead person has come back to haunt them. Visitation dreams are recorded throughout history.[20] There may be a spiritual dimension in visitation dreams that brings solace since they show an afterlife in which the dead live on. As Kelly Bulkeley and Patricia Bulkley observe, "Visitation dreams do not deny death so much as transcend it, providing experiential evidence of human connections that extend beyond the end of mortal life."[21]

Many children see visitation dreams as a form of communication. Such dreams deliver messages, provide advice, or give warnings. They may offer forgiveness or reassurance and clarity to a child who is confused about the circumstances of the death. In their intensity, visitation dreams can have a life-altering impact on the dreamer. They may bring about a change of perspective including spiritual change.[22]

Justine, aged 15, told me about her vivid dream:

In reality my father died nearly six years ago of leukemia. I dreamt not long ago that the doorbell rang and he was standing on the doorstep with all his cases ready to come home.

Her dream can also be described as a wish-fulfillment dream. In reality, she knows her father will never come back to live in her home but she feels he is still part of her world. Chrissy, aged 11, recounts a similar dream:

It was Christmas and my Nana had already died but all my family go to her house for Christmas dinner. We all sat at the table and Nana's space was left empty. After dinner we all opened our presents and left Nana's armchair empty. Then my Nana appears in the space left and talks to us all about Christmas then she says goodbye and disappears.

When I asked Chrissy what the dream meant to her she said, "I think my Nana was trying to say goodbye." She felt comforted by the dream and thought that, even though her grandmother was dead, she was still part of the family. Such a view reflects the significance of continuing bonds in the grieving process.

Spiritual Dimension

In cultures throughout the world dreaming is thought to connect both the past and the future. Australian Aborigines believe that life and death are part of a cycle that begins and ends in dreamtime and that as we dream we are liberated from the limitations of time and space. Ancestors visit in dreams and bring wisdom and knowledge to the dreamer. The Narranga-ga tribe say that the human spirit can leave the dreamer's body and travel and make contact with other spirits, including those of the dead. The Jupagalk Aboriginals believe that a person who is sick can be helped by the visit of a dead relative. Those continuing bonds bring aid and succor.[23]

Swiss psychiatrist C. G. Jung observed that many "big" or numinous dreams occur in childhood. These are those dreams that stay with you throughout your life and may be life changing. They have a felt power, intensity, and vividness that profoundly impacts on the dreamer. Jung emphasized the psychological and spiritual importance of these dreams, calling them "the richest jewels in the treasure house of psychic experience."[24]

For some children, dreams bring them closer to the sacred and the transcendent that can inspire and guide them through the healing process. They provide comfort, especially when a random event such as manslaughter or a road traffic collision has caused the death. Where the dead person is cared for by God or angels or other important spiritual beings in dreams, it can ease the grief of a bereaved child. Fifteen-year-old Aidan said, "After my father died, I dreamt of a big hand coming down out of the sky and I knew it was God showing me that I would be taken care of and that He was taking care of my father." We need to take into account the faith, spirituality, and the beliefs of young people when we work with their dreams.

Sometimes dreams have insights or knowledge of future events. Eleven-year-old Aloysius recounted his dream:

Just one week before my grandma died I had a very strange dream. I dreamt I was walking down the backs of some houses and I found a memory card of a man. I picked it up, carried on walking and came to a back garden. In this back garden there was my grandma with a tall dark man in a black cloak and a black hat. They were at a man's wake and it was the same man as in the memory card. The next week my grandma died. She had a wake and I was given a memory card of her.

Memory cards, commonly used in Irish communities, carry a photograph of the dead person, details of their life and a prayer to be said for the repose of their soul. Aloysius thought his dream was about an impending death but did not connect it with his grandmother, who was well at the time. The memory card, the wake, and the black clothes reinforce the death imagery.

Children sometimes dream about their own death as Vivienne, aged 13, told me:

I was in hospital and the doctors were operating on me and my spirit rose right out of my body and my spirit was looking right down on me. My body was dead but my spirit was alive trying to wake my body up and when my spirit returned to my body I felt the bed shake and woke up.

This was Vivienne's first dream of an out-of-body experience and confirmed her belief that our spirit or soul lives on after death.

There has been much written about the area of psychic phenomena and dreams but children are often unwilling to talk about them in case they are disbelieved or ridiculed.[25] Anna dreams about future events mainly concerning her family. She only talks to her father about them because: "He is the only one who takes me seriously about my forward-in-time dreams."

One of the most famous precognitive dreams in childhood relating to death is that of Eryl Mai Jones. Ten-year-old Eryl woke up and insisted that her mother listen to her dream even though her mother said she was too busy. Eryl persisted and told her mother that she dreamed that something black came over the school and completely covered it. She was so disturbed by the dream that she said she did not want to go to school. Eventually, her mother's will prevailed and Eryl went to school on that fateful day when, with 143 fellow students, she died. Her school in Aberfan was buried under a mountain of coal slurry.[26]

Dying children sometimes speak of relatives who are waiting for them "on the other side." As Elisabeth Kubler-Ross, who worked extensively with children on the cusp of death, says, "... every single child who mentioned that someone was waiting for them mentioned a person who had actually preceded them in death, even if by only a few moments. And yet none of these children had been informed of the recent death of the relatives by us at any time."[27] She firmly believed that dreams of the dead are contacts on a spiritual plane.[28]

The week after Elise, aged nine, had spoken to me of her dreams, she brought me a drawing she had done at home. At the top it said, "To Brenda, this is the angel I sometimes see in my dreams. She is called Angel Topia, and sometimes she says she loves me very much and is always protecting me and will always be my Guardian Angel." Below was a picture of a smiling angel with a dress covered with diamonds and hearts and a pair of wings with shining diamonds blazing out. The joy this angel gave to Elise was so moving for me to witness and obviously a great comfort to the bereaved child.

How Do You Draw Heaven?

Paul was an eight-year-old pupil at a school for children with special educational needs when his grandfather died. In school, the day after the death, he was very upset and one of the nonteaching assistants took him to one side and during their conversation reassured him that it was normal to be upset when someone you loved died. When he returned to class, at his teacher's suggestion, he drew himself with his granddad in the park. Then he said, "I don't really know how to draw heaven but I think it's a big city on top of a cloud. God lives in the church and the people live together in houses on the green hills. It is always sunny." He also wrote, "I loved my granddad very much. I will miss him. He has gone to heaven. He will be happy. He will be watching me."

A Practical Guide for Helping a Child Who Has Disturbing Dreams or Nightmares

- Listen to the story of the dream.
- Do not judge the content of the dream. Dreams are not "right" or "wrong"; they are expressions of the inner world of the child.
- Value the dream. Do not dismiss the dream as silly or unimportant.
- Encourage the child to tell you what the dream means to him. Do not put your interpretation on the dream.
- Reassure the child that her disturbing dreams do not mean she is crazy. Help her to realize that dreams are a way of dealing with her loss.
- Ask supportive, open questions to explore the dream: How did you feel in the dream? What was the happiest part of the meeting in the dream?
- Allow the child to go at his own pace: do not force him to go on talking when he wants to stop.
- Help the child to make links to waking events. If she was chased by a monster can she think of a time when she was chased, and if so who was chasing her?

- Respect the child's confidentiality. Do not talk about the child's dream unless you have his permission.

Make a Dream Catcher

Dream catchers originated in North America where First Nation Natives constructed a circle with a web of threads across it and included decorative beads and feathers. They believed that the dream catcher trapped bad dreams and nightmares and acted as a protective amulet. In making a dream catcher with a child you have the opportunity to talk about dreams and how they feature in the child's life.

Sally, an eight-year-old girl, was having difficulty sleeping after the murder of her sister. She had a recurring nightmare of her sister: she knew her sister was there but could not see her face and this terrified her. None of the professionals who were supporting her following the murder asked her about how she slept or about her dreams. Finally, a dream therapist helped Sally and her mother to talk about her dreams, to draw them and to make a dream catcher and Sally was able to move on from her "stuck" grieving position.[29]

Create a New Movie

The creativity of children is a joy. You can use it to work on dreams as if they were films. The dreamer is the director of the dream movie, the actors, the set designer, the lighting technician, the makeup artist, the location scout; in fact, the dreamer can be everything. Ask the dreamer about the actors. Who are they and are they just right for the film or does he need other people; if so, who? Whatever he wants to change or develop in the dream, he can. This technique can be used playfully or seriously depending on the needs and maturity of the child.

This technique can also be very useful in giving children the opportunity to be superheroes in their own dreams. Anything is possible: They can fly away from danger, enlist the help of huge creatures that obey their commands, they can become invisible or all-powerful. In their dream movies they can tap into their own creativity and strengths and transform distressing dreams into positive experiences.

Finally, what bereaved children need is care, consistency, kindness and compassion. If you can provide those qualities children will learn to trust you and enable you to help them through one of the most significant events in their life. The life of a child who has been bereaved has been changed irrevocably but you can foster resilience by working on those dreams that both distress and empower. Be tender—in sharing dreams we share our deepest selves.

Notes

1. Brenda Mallon, *Working with Bereaved Children and Young People* (London: Sage, 2011).

2. Brenda Mallon, *Children Dreaming: Pictures in My Pillow* (London: Penguin, 1989).

3. Ibid., 11.

4. J. William Worden, *Children and Grief: When a Parent Dies* (New York: The Guilford Press, 1996), 29.

5. Colin Murray Parkes, "Bereavement as a Psychosocial Transition: Processes of Adaptation to Change," *Journal of Social Issues* 44, no. 3 (1988): 53–65.

6. Robert A. Neimeyer, "Grief, Loss and the Quest for Meaning: Narrative Contributions to Bereavement Care," *Bereavement Care* 24, no. 2 (2005): 27–29.

7. Edna St. Vincent Millay, *Letters of Edna St Vincent Millay* (New York: Harpers, 1915).

8. Dennis Klass, Phyllis R. Silverman, and Steven L. Nickman (Eds.), *Continuing Bonds: New Understandings of Grief* (London: Taylor & Francis, 1996).

9. D. G. LoConto, "Death and Dreams: A Sociological Approach to Grieving and Identity," *Omega* 37, 1998: 171–185.

10. Catherine A. Cooper, "Children's Dreams during the Grief Process," *Professional School of Counselling* 3, no. 2 (1999): 137–140.

Mary C. Cogar and Clara E. Hill, "Examining the Effects of Brief Individual Dream Interpretation," *Dreaming* 2, no. 4 (1992): 239–248.

11. Matthew Arnold, "Faded Leaves" (1855) no. 5. (First published in 1852 as "Longing.")

12. Gordon Riches and Pamela Dawson, *An Intimate Loneliness: Supporting Bereaved Parents and Siblings* (Buckinghamshire: Open University Press, 2000): 37.

13. Phyllis R. Silverman, Steven L. Nickman, and J. William Worden, "Detachment Revisited: The Child's Reconstruction of a Dead Parent," *American Journal of Orthopsychiatry* 62, no. 4 (1992): 494–503.

14. Mallon, *Children Dreaming*.

15. Dennis Klass, Phyllis R. Silverman, and Steven L. Nickman (Eds.), *Continuing Bonds: New Understandings of Grief* (London: Taylor & Francis, 1996).

16. Silverman et al., "Child's Reconstruction," 497.

17. Brenda Mallon, *Dream Time with Children: Learning to Dream, Dreaming to Learn* (London: Jessica Kingsley, 2002).

18. D. Schuurman, "Invited Speaker: Valerie Maasdorp on Resiliency in Palliative Care," The Forum 34, nos. 3 & 9 (2008): 4.

19. John Donne, *Elegy 10 "The Dream,"* Selected Poems (London: Orion Publishing Group, 1997), 56.

20. Kate Adams and Brendan Hyde, *The Spiritual Dimension of Childhood* (London: Jessica Kingsley, 2008).

Mallon, *Bereaved Children*.

Kelly Bulkeley, Transforming Dreams: Learning Spiritual Lessons from the Dreams You Never Forget (New York: Wiley, 2000).

21. Kelly Bulkeley and Patricia M. Bulkley, *Dreaming Beyond Death: A Guide to Pre-Death Dreams and Visions* (Boston: Beacon Press, 2005).

22. Jennifer E. Shorter, "Visitation Dreams in Grieving Individuals: A Phenomenological Inquiry into the Relationship between Dreams and the Grieving Process," *Institute of Transpersonal Psychology,* Dissertation, 183 pages; publication number 3397063 (2010).

23. Richard Lansdown, "Fourth International Conference on Children and Death, Editorial," *Bereavement Care* 18, no. 3 (1999): 43–45.

24. Alan Siegel and Kelly Bulkeley, *Dream Catching: Every Parent's Guide to Exploring and Understanding Children's Dreams and Nightmares* (New York: Three Rivers Press, 1998).

25. Mallon, *Children Dreaming.*

Aileen H. Cooke, *Out of the Mouth of Babes: ESP in Children* (London: James Clarke & Co., 1968).

26. John C. Barker, "Premonitions of the Aberfan Disaster," *Journal of the Society of Psychical Research* 44 (1967): 169–181.

27. Elisabeth Kubler-Ross, *On Children and Death* (New York: Collier Books, 1983), 110.

28. Elisabeth Kubler-Ross, *Death, the Final Stage of Growth* (New York: Prentice Hall, 1975).

29. Ruth Harrison, *Working with Homicide*, Presentation to the Manchester Area Bereavement Conference (2000).

Bibliography

Adams, Kate and Brendan Hyde. *The Spiritual Dimension of Childhood*. London: Jessica Kingsley, 2008.

Arnold, Matthew. "Faded Leaves." (1855) No. 5. (First published in 1852 as "Longing.")

Barker, John C. "Premonitions of the Aberfan Disaster." *Journal of the Society of Psychical Research* 44, 1967: 169–81.

Bulkeley, Kelly. *Transforming Dreams: Learning Spiritual Lessons from the Dreams You Never Forget.* New York: Wiley, 2000.

Bulkeley, Kelly. "Big Dreams in Childhood: The Richest Jewels in the Treasure House of Psychic Experience." retrieved May 6, 2015, 14:18. http://www.huffingtonpost.com/kelly-bulkeley-phd/big-dreams_b_2761411.html (2013).

Bulkeley, Kelly and Patricia M. Bulkley. *Children's Dreams: Understanding the Most Memorable Dreams and Nightmares of Childhood.* Lanham, Maryland: Rowan & Littlefield, 2012.

Bulkeley, Kelly and Patricia M. Bulkley. *Dreaming beyond Death: A Guide to Pre-Death Dreams and Visions.* Boston: Beacon Press, 2005.

Cooke, Aileen H. *Out of the Mouth of Babes: ESP in Children.* London: James Clarke & Co., 1968.

Cooper, Catherine A. "Children's Dreams during the Grief Process." *Professional School of Counselling* 3, no. 2 (1999): 137–140.

Cogar, Mary C. and Clara E. Hill. "Examining the Effects of Brief Individual Dream Interpretation." *Dreaming* 2, no. 4 (1992): 239–248.

Donne, John. *Elegy 10 "The Dream," Selected Poems.* London: Orion Publishing Group, 1997.

Harrison, Ruth. *Working with Homicide.* Presentation to the Manchester Area Bereavement Conference, 2000.

Jung, C. G. *Dreams, Memories and Reflections.* New York: Vintage, 1990.

Klass, Dennis, Phyllis R. Silverman, and Steven L. Nickman (Eds.). *Continuing Bonds: New Understandings of Grief.* London: Taylor & Francis, 1996.

Kubler-Ross, Elisabeth. *Death, the Final Stage of Growth.* New York: Prentice Hall, 1975.

Kubler-Ross, Elisabeth. *On Children and Death.* New York: Collier Books, 1983.

Lansdown, Richard. "Fourth International Conference on Children and Death, Editorial." *Bereavement Care* 18, no. 3 (1999): 43–45.

Lewis, Clive Staples. *A Grief Observed.* London: Faber and Faber Ltd., 1966.

LoConto, D. G. Death and Dreams: a Sociological Approach to Grieving and Identity. *Omega,* 37 (1998): 171–185.

Mallon, Brenda. *Children Dreaming: Pictures in My Pillow.* London: Penguin, 1989.

Mallon, Brenda. *Dreams, Counselling and Healing.* Dublin: Gill & Macmillan, 2000.

Mallon, Brenda. *Dream Time with Children: Learning to Dream, Dreaming to Learn.* London: Jessica Kingsley, 2002.

Mallon, Brenda. "Dreams and Bereavement." *Bereavement Care* 24, no. 3 (2005): 43–46.

Mallon, Brenda. *Working with Bereaved Children and Young People.* London: Sage, 2011.

Millay, Edna St. Vincent. *Letters of Edna St. Vincent Millay.* New York: Harpers, 1915.

Neimeyer, Robert A. "Grief, Loss and the Quest for Meaning: Narrative Contributions to Bereavement Care." *Bereavement Care* 24, no. 2 (2005): 27–29.

Parkes, Colin, Murray. "Bereavement as a Psychosocial Transition: Processes of Adaptation to Change." *Journal of Social Issues* 44, no. 3 (1988): 53–65.

Prasad, Jamuna and Ian Stevenson. "A Survey of Spontaneous Psychical Experiences in School Children of Uttar Pradesh India." *International Journal of Parapsychology* 10, 1968: 241–261.

Riches, Gordon and Pamela Dawson. *An Intimate Loneliness: Supporting Bereaved Parents and Siblings.* Buckinghamshire: Open University Press, 2000.

Schuurman, D. "Invited Speaker: Valerie Maasdorp on Resiliency in Palliative Care." *The Forum* 34, no. 3 (2008): 9.

Siegel, Alan and Kelly Bulkeley. *Dream Catching: Every Parent's Guide to Exploring and Understanding Children's Dreams and Nightmares.* MA: Three Rivers Press, 1998.

Shorter, Jennifer E. "Visitation Dreams in Grieving Individuals: A Phenomenological Inquiry into the Relationship between Dreams and the Grieving Process." *Institute of Transpersonal Psychology.* Dissertation, 183 pages; publication number 3397063, 2010.

Silverman, Phyllis R., Steven L. Nickman, and J. William Worden. "Detachment Revisited: The Child's Reconstruction of a Dead Parent." *American Journal of Orthopsychiatry* 62, no. 4 (1992): 494–503.

Worden, J. W. *Children and Grief: When a Parent Dies.* New York: The Guilford Press, 1996.

CHAPTER TEN

Weirdness in the Night: Terrors and Disorders in Children's Sleep

Ryan Hurd

When my daughter's sleep terrors first began, I made a few missteps. I did not realize what was happening, so I dealt with her as if she was awake. One time, she was crying in her bed. I went in, curled up next to her, and asked her what was wrong over and over. I was terrified by the idea that my daughter would be filled with such anguish that she would wake in the middle of the night and cry. "What could be wrong with her?" I asked. It seemed like something terrible must be going on. But nothing panned out over the following days, and I was reminded of the strong emotions that accompanied my own night terrors when I was a child.

Noelle, mother of Mia, age 9

Noelle's account of trying to comfort her daughter brings to the surface the real desperation that millions of parents feel around the world every single night. Sleep troubles and bizarre dream experiences, which I am calling "weirdness in the night," are quite common but few of us have been taught what the causes of these ailments are, when they are dangerous and when not to worry, and, most importantly, *what to do* when they erupt out of the stillness of an ordinary school night.

This chapter addresses common varieties of children's night weirdness—known by sleep doctors as *parasomnias*. The American Academy of Sleep Medicine defines parasomnias as "abnormal sleep related movements, behaviors, perceptions, dreams and autonomous nervous system activity."[1] Or, as parents might describe it: the sudden flailing and screaming nonstop in the middle of the night, the walking around like zombies, unresponsive and impervious to reason, and the repetitive nightmares that invariably end with a shivering child spending the rest of the night in the big bed. While often normal and not health threatening, these events can be exhausting and nerve-racking for parents and caregivers. As someone who has experienced several of these parasomnias in childhood, I would also add *soul-rending* to the list of descriptors. I personally suffered from all sorts of night weirdness, culminating at age 14 with the hyperrealistic vision of being held down in bed by an evil force that tried to crush the air out of my lungs with invisible hands. That experience in particular, which I now know to be a textbook example of isolated sleep paralysis, kick-started my lifelong interest in dreams, nightmares, and unusual vision states. Now a parent myself, I am experiencing the night weirdness in a new role, and am thankful to have at least some clue to what is going on with these hidden aspects of the night that are so infrequently discussed in polite society.

This chapter provides current research, preventative measures, and practical ways for understanding and working with children's parasomnias. Similar to dreamwork, acknowledging parasomnias provides a window into the interior lives of children, giving caregivers a chance to openly honor the deeper messages and opportunities nested within these truly weird episodes of the night. In many cases, children's night weirdness is not dangerous and simply requires patience, a comforting presence in the moment, and preparation of some protective actions. Still, these events can sometimes be considered red flags for more serious issues that require medical attention. Often, an eruption in night weirdness can be managed by improving sleep health, especially reducing sleep debt and identifying more serious sleep issues. Lastly, mindfully turning the gaze toward caregivers' own lifestyle profiles, stress management, and relational tensions, with a sincere willingness to make meaningful changes, can also positively affect children's sleep eruptions in the night.

Primary parasomnias are generally grouped into sleep–wake transition disorders, NREM arousal disorders, and REM parasomnias. Covered in detail in this chapter are the last two of these categories, including: sleepwalking, night terrors, and sleep paralysis visions. Although other sleep behaviors will also be addressed, such as nightmare disorders, this chapter is not meant to be an exhaustive list of sleep troubles in children, or to be taken as a clinical sourcebook, but rather as a starting point for surveying the landscape of children's "weirdness in the night," especially at the crossroads of sleep troubles and dreaming.

Unfortunately, unlike ordinary dreams and nightmares, many parasomnias are not clearly remembered afterwards, so common dreamwork techniques are not effective. Many occurrences of parasomnias are simply a part of the maturation of the human brain and cannot be prevented. Events that are remembered, such as nightmares and sleep paralysis visions in teens, can be worked with using dreamwork techniques such as art play, dream theater and other fun methods that honor the dream's depth and simultaneously strengthen the child's resilience.[2] Before we look at the solutions to children's most common sleep weirdness, let us frame the social backdrop to children's sleep in the twenty-first century.

Good Sleep Is Not Guaranteed

Our children's sleep is disturbed, perhaps now more than ever before. When sleep is restricted, quality of health is compromised, increasing the risk of serious illness such as obesity and diabetes. With this generalized risk, of course, parasomnias and other sleep symptoms are more likely. Many adults find it easy to forego getting enough sleep themselves, yet a public health crisis has been quietly building as children and teens emulate their role models by entering into the twenty-first century culture of 24/7 workaholism, media consumption, and wireless social connectivity.

In brief, here is a rundown of the largest issues facing children's sleep health today:

- In general, children are not getting enough sleep. School age children need 9–11 hours of sleep, but are getting closer to 5–6.[3] Teens need 8–10 hours of sleep a night, but on average are getting 7.5 hours a night.[4]
- Children are staying up later and watching more media. Forty-three percent of school-aged children have a TV in the bedroom.[5] Seventy-seven percent of teens (ages 13–18) are looking at a computer monitor the hour before bedtime.[6] Recent studies suggest that kids with TVs or computers in the bedroom watch an hour more media, and get 30 minutes less sleep a night than those children who sleep in a monitor-free bedroom.[7]
- Children's sleep is being increasingly interrupted by technology, too. Sixty percent of adolescents and teens use mobile devices after "lights out."[8] Eighteen percent of teens are awoken by cell phone calls, e-mails, and texts several times a week.[9] Use of mobile devices after lights out is related to many sleep problems, including: short sleep duration, subjective poor sleep quality, excessive daytime sleepiness, and insomnia symptoms.[10]
- After late nights consisting of poor and interrupted sleep, children are waking up too early because most schools start early in the morning. In the United States, the nationwide average is 8:03 a.m.[11] Most pediatricians and sleep professionals suggest that children's sleep rhythm is naturally weighted toward later bed times and sleeping in past daybreak. In fact, the American Academy of Sleep Medicine, the Center for Disease Control, and the

American Academy of Pediatrics support later start time for schools, especially for teens.[12] The situation is similar in the United Kingdom and Europe, where some limited successes for later school start times have recently been established.[13]

Reviewing the social backdrop for children's sleep health is especially relevant for preventing the triggers that lead to parasomnias and terrifying night hallucinations. Electronic devices and new media consumption patterns are not harmless, or simply this generation's version of reading a comic book by flashlight after lights-out. The blue light from electronic devices delays the release of melatonin into the bloodstream, preventing drowsiness, delayed sleep as well as restful sleep throughout the night.[14] Interrupted sleep, also known as sleep fragmentation, can be as damaging as not getting enough sleep for children.[15] Some effects include daytime sleepiness, worsened mood, and mental decline. Taken together, these effects have inspired researchers to use a new term for modern sleep habits that include media use before bed: *junk sleep*.[16]

As we shall see, the antidote is providing parents and caregivers with the vocabulary of improving *sleep hygiene*, which can be defined as the practices that protect and maintain healthy sleeping conditions. That is just the surface, though. Sleep hygiene is really more than changing overt behaviors. An integrative sleep medicine perspective also includes the importance of cultural attitudes and even spiritual dimensions for healthy sleep. As individuals, we may have to dig deep to discover our biases against healthy sleep, as Western culture does not promote the importance of sleep for health and wellness.

Psychologist Rubin Naiman suggests:

> Our struggle with night is ultimately a struggle with denied aspects of our own darkness. Confusing the literal darkness of night with the metaphoric darkness of life, we blindly project our feelings about the latter onto the former. We then mitigate our fear of darkness through the excessive use of evening light, effectively extending daytime's custody over us deep into the night and seriously eroding our *night consciousness*. Indoors and out, our nights are lit up beyond reason—so far beyond what necessity and safety might dictate. Like a frightened child, the planet sleeps with its lights on. In the end, sleep and dream disorders are largely symptomatic of this deeper fear of night and its damaging segregation from day.[17]

In line with Dr. Naiman's analysis, the aim of this chapter is to not only address tactics and solutions for children's sleep disturbances but also help revitalize the importance of night consciousness for modern life. Again, this chapter will not cover all of the sleep disorders (currently 26 and growing), but rather the most common ones that plague children's sleep and their caregiver's sleep as well. The first category of parasomnias discussed are a category of sleep disorders known as NREM arousal disorders. These behaviors are not considered primary sleep "diseases," such as narcolepsy or sleep apnea, but rather as disorders in which partial waking arousal disturbs the normal staging of sleep.[18] By definition, these disorders are associated with NREM sleep, which includes light sleep (N1-N2) as well as deep sleep (N3). Sleepwalking and sleep terrors are two of the most common NREM arousal disorders in children. Two REM parasomnias will then be discussed: nightmares and sleep paralysis.

Sleepwalking

> When I was a kid, I did a lot of yelling in my sleep, pounding walls, and walking into other rooms. I said a lot of ludicrous things. Allegedly, I once pounded on the wall in my bedroom and when my parents came in, I exasperatedly explained that "It wouldn't lay down!" I learned that my parents would just turn me around, tell me it was time to go to sleep, and that I would go. (Noelle, Philadelphia)

Sleepwalking, or somnambulism, is very common in children. Generally occurring between the ages of 4 and 12, sleepwalking happens occasionally for about 20 percent of children, and more frequently in about 3–4 percent of children.[19] Most children outgrow the condition, which peaks around 11–12 years old, although 25 percent of sleepwalking children still do it in adulthood.[20] Sleepwalking erupts out of deep sleep, when delta waves predominate the sleeping brain in the first half of the night. Sleepwalking and other arousal disorders usually surface within an hour or two after the child goes to sleep. The sleepwalker rouses and moves about for a few minutes with open but distant eyes. Children can perform complex behavior as well, although their movements may be clumsy and not well defined. When confronted, a sleepwalker may simply navigate around the obstacle without acknowledgment or respond foggily at best. If left alone, they generally go back to bed or another place they habitually rest, such as a couch in the living room or their parent's bedroom.[21] According to the National Sleep Foundation, the best course of action for parents is to wake the child and gently lead them back to bed in order to prevent any injuries.[22]

Sleepwalking can run in the family.[23] In a recent study, researchers found that "children with one parent with a history of sleepwalking had three times the odds of becoming a sleepwalker, and children with both parents with a history had seven times the odds."[24] Myths passed down through the generations are common, and parents are likely to follow folk advice, such as the old wives' tale that it is dangerous or unlucky to wake a sleepwalker. Actually, waking the sleeper can prevent injury. The "micro-culture" of sleep habits that is passed down through the family line can also provide emotional support. For example, Philadelphia resident and parent Noelle, who also sleepwalked as a child, suggested that her mother's advice provided her with comfort when she shared her own children's sleep troubles. "Because we talked so much about my sleep behavior, I already knew some strategies for coping. I also knew what didn't work."[25]

For those who are prone to sleepwalking, episodes can be triggered when a child is sleep deprived, ill from a cold, or physically exhausted. A pattern of an inconsistent sleep schedule can also trigger the symptom. In general, stress and anxiety play major roles. Beware: medications may also have an effect; there are too many to list but common ones include over-the-counter allergy medications and cough syrups. Children with chronic sleepwalking often also have other sleep symptoms such as sleep-obstructed breathing and restless leg syndrome, in which case the sleepwalking may be a red flag for a larger health concern.[26]

Interpreting and Working with Sleepwalking

One of the enduring mysteries about sleepwalking is the question of how meaningful the sleepwalker's actions are. Children's acts can seem purposeful and even goal-oriented at times, such as opening and unlocking doors, and urinating in inappropriate places. Later, sleepwalkers usually do not remember the episode at all, or only faintly. However eerie this may seem, the prevailing theory is that children's actions while sleepwalking are most likely habitual activities that could be considered a form of automatism.[27] Sleepwalking is not "dream walking." However, this is not to say that children's behaviors during sleepwalking are necessarily random. Going even further, dreamworker Jeremy Taylor notes that some children's actions during sleepwalking could be seen as "involuntary theater," in which they perform activities that might be charged or significant for adults in the house.[28] Although his evidence is anecdotal, Taylor's suggestion can at least be considered a worthy hypothesis, as sleep specialists in general do not look to psychological patterns when treating sleep disturbances, but rather focus on managing and preventing future episodes. An exception to this trend is research into the sleepwalking of trauma survivors, which suggests that in some cases, sleepwalking might indeed include dissociative behaviors that are usually "kept in check" during the day.[29] Formally called *compensation*, this theory of a nighttime "relief valve" opens the discussion to more sophisticated interpretations of sleepwalking behavior, although much more research is needed in terms of the value of psychological treatment for parasomnias in general.

More important is that children are safe, and that precautions are taken to protect frequent sleepwalkers. Indeed, newspapers are full of stories of children who have been injured due to somnambulism. Adolescents and teens tend to travel farther than young children in their sleepwalking, so the risk of injury is greater for them. In 2009, for example, *The Daily Mail* reported that a teenager plunged 25 feet after walking through an open window while sleepwalking. In this case, the lucky teen landed in the grass below and reported no injuries.[30] In another case, a four-year-old Norwegian girl sleepwalked for three miles in the snow wearing only her underclothes and boots. She also lucked out, as she was found by local villagers who quickly took her inside and called the authorities.[31]

Like many of the NREM arousal disorders, sleepwalking requires simple, but often inconvenient, precautions once caregivers are surprised with the first episode. Some lock interior doors at night, including the child's bedroom door. Locks that the child never opens on their own, such as eyehook locks out of their reach, are preferable because sleepwalkers can habitually do many complex things. Secure dangerous objects, and clear obstacles in the home so there are clear paths. Consider blocking staircases at night with a safety gate. If sleepwalking becomes frequent and is also paired with other sleep troubles such as night terrors or excessive daytime sleepiness, consult a medical provider.

When sleepwalking rears, also consider the atmosphere of the house and even your own stress levels, as tension and anxiety are easily absorbed by children. Busy lives are a guarantee, but stressful times call for proactive measures, such as taking time for stress reduction techniques. The goal is to induce the *relaxation response* (RR), which has been clinically documented to have a powerful effect on our minds and bodies. Its short-term effects include improving mood and metabolism while reducing anxiety, muscle tension, and sleep troubles. Long-term benefits include slowing the aging process and reducing the risk of major disease.[32] The good news is that this ancient antidote to stress usually requires only 10–15 minutes of our time. Walking in nature, gardening, bathing, reading, sharing memories, and taking care of a pet are all wonderful ways to relax together.

Equally important is establishing an evening routine that works with, rather than against, natural sleep patterns. Limit media consumption in the evenings and especially limit the close use of monitors, tablets and phones due to the sleep-disrupting effects of blue light. Rubin Naiman suggests that honoring dusk can have a profound effect as well.[33] Rather than turning on bright lights as the sun goes down, allow the house to have reduced lighting for an hour before the child's bedtime. Simulate dusk if need be, with the use of light-blocking curtains and shades. Consider bedtime not as a dividing line that is rushed toward as one more task to be overcome, but a slow transition that begins with dim lighting and relaxation. Spiritual practices, such as prayer, gratitude exercises, and meditation can also be easily incorporated into bedtime rituals, as they not only support the RR, but also enable deep bonding with children at a time when they are often feeling vulnerable.

The preferred clinical treatment of sleepwalking, as well as sleep terrors, is a technique called "scheduled awakening." Parents are instructed to take notes of the general time when the sleepwalking occurs, and then wake up the child 15–20 minutes before the event time for an entire month.[34]

Sleep Terrors

The memory of my own childhood sleep terror from age eight or nine involves "waking up" in my parents' bedroom while they comforted me. I had apparently run into their room screaming and was inconsolable for several minutes. I recall a vague but intense feeling of having been in an infinite space where gray colored pillars, extending infinitely up and down, moved around me. There was a terrible feeling of deep loneliness, of infinite emptiness and of a vast, unfeeling and mechanistic universe. I felt very small. But the most haunting aspect of the experience was the lingering emotional residue after the event. I was not swayed by my parents' reassurances that "it was just a dream," but I was certainly comforted by their closeness and soothing voices.

Better known as "night terrors," and classically defined as *pavor nocturnus*, this parasomnia is an arousal disorder associated with deep sleep that generally arises within the first 90 minutes of going to bed. However, these terrors can come during daytime naps as well, leading prominent researchers to support the more general term *sleep terrors*.[35] Sleep terror prevalence peaks at 1.5 years but phases out by age 12–14.[36] Whenever they occur, sleep terrors are recognized instantly because the child suddenly screams out loud, often flailing around with a look of terror. The child is inconsolable for several minutes, and does not acknowledge anyone despite sitting up in bed with open eyes. Sometimes, the child will run about as if trying to escape; these episodes therefore can be accompanied by sleepwalking, but are much more frantic and dangerous than sleepwalking alone due to the erratic behavior. Other times, the child may seem catatonic with fear, trembling, sweating while staring blankly. Sleep terrors are usually not remembered—the emotional atmosphere usually carries over without dream images, although my own numerous experiences show that some people may be more likely than others to remember their night terrors. Disturbing for everyone involved, most sleep terrors are nonetheless benign and simply a part of childhood development, like sleepwalking and other NREM arousal disorders. However, if night terrors and sleepwalking are frequent, the likelihood increases of a deeper sleep health issue, such as restless leg syndrome or sleep-disordered breathing.[37]

Sleep terrors are often confused with other forms of night weirdness such as nightmares and sleep paralysis visions. Although terrifying to experience and difficult to watch someone go through, it is important to acknowledge that sleep terrors are not bad dreams. In fact, sleep terrors occur as a fugue of arousal from deep sleep, not REM sleep, which is the state associated with both nightmares and sleep paralysis.

Interpreting and Working with Sleep Terrors

This arousal disorder does not generally include recalled dream content and so they cannot generally be interpreted as dreams. Still, like sleepwalking, their sudden and repetitive occurrence can serve as a red flag for the deterioration of sleep health as well as insufficient stress management. Note that pervasive snoring or mouth breathing during sleep in association with increased sleep terrors could indicate developing sleep apnea. Parents take note: teens who begin having routine sleep terrors, with or without aggravated sleepwalking, have higher risks for mental illness, and may also be harboring substance abuse issues.

Similar to sleepwalking and other arousal disorders, most of the time sleep terrors cannot be fully prevented so much as successfully managed. For children, the best scenario is to be at the child's side once the terror begins, or as quickly as possible, in order to prevent injury. Soothe the child primarily with words until she comes out of the fugue. Once the child is cognizant, physical comforting will be more effective. In my estimation, treating the sleep terror as a primary experience, with respect for the child's emotional state, rather than quick dismissal as "just a dream," goes a long way. Let the child know he or she is safe. Acknowledging fear by emphasizing safety provides an anchor to the present moment. Susie Parker, a Certified Pediatric Sleep Specialist based in Chicago, Illinois, suggests, "When the night terror is over, it's a good idea to use soothing, relaxing words, like 'Go back to sleep, I'm here to keep you safe,' to just lull your child back into their bed to continue their sleep."[38]

As with sleepwalking, night terrors are triggered through elevated levels of stress and anxiety as well as sleep restriction. For this reason, they tend to come at times of life's crossroads and transitions, such as moving house or starting school. Stress at the family level is no doubt high at this time, as children absorb and respond to the tension expressed by caregivers. While stress cannot be eliminated at times such as these, it can be managed proactively. Parents will find that attending to their own anxiety is as important as providing comforting structure for the child during these times. When night terrors erupt, ask, "What can I do to better incorporate stress relief into our lives?" Establishing strong sleep patterns with a patterned bedtime routine is also critical for children suffering from sleep terrors, as well as eliminating sleep stealers such as computer and mobile technology use after dinner.

Jeremy Taylor notes that sleep terrors may provide a window into the existential fears of a child, and may also reflect a "spiritual vacuum" in the household. Similar to his interpretation of sleep walking, the sleep terror represents "an unconscious (and thus involuntary) request that the people who are awake to see and respond to the theater of profound terror and distress will 'get it' what a terrible situation the lack of spoken clarity about deepest (religious/spiritual) beliefs, suspicions and experiences is for the dreamer. Usually this is something the dreamer is not even fully conscious of when awake."[39]

Nightmare Disorders

Every child has a bad dream every once in a while. Like sleep terrors and sleepwalking, the occasional nightmare is a part of growing up. But some children suffer even more, and their nightmares affect their daytime mood and energy. An estimated 5 percent of children suffer from nightmares at least once a week.[40] When nightmares are persistent, disturbing a child's sleep regularly and having a strong effect on day-to-day life, a diagnosis of nightmare disorder may be given by a sleep specialist or psychiatrist and treated clinically with a combination of psychotherapy and pharmaceuticals. Children who have been traumatized, due to abuse, witnessing extreme violence, or surviving a natural disaster, also have frequent, repetitive nightmares that realistically replay the traumatic event. These children may be suffering from acute stress reactions; if diagnosed with post-traumatic stress disorder, they can be treated clinically with a variety of nightmare therapy techniques.[41]

From the perspective of integrative sleep science, persistent nightmares should first and foremost be treated as a parasomnia that has biological roots as well as psychological correlations. This means first attending to all the triggers of poor sleep that have been discussed previously with regard to sleep terrors and sleepwalking. Junk sleep, not enough regularity in sleep, and not enough sleep in general can trigger nightmares due to the effects of bodily stress on sleep staging throughout the night. Like NREM parasomnias, nightmares are not uncommon during stressful times such as divorce and settling into a new neighborhood.[42] These are the times to secure a child's environment, both physically and emotionally, and be proactive about incorporating healthy (and fun) stress reduction activities into the day-to-day schedule.

Sleep Paralysis

When I was 14 years old, I recorded the following dream and waking experience in my brand new dream journal:

> I'm standing around and the phone rings. I went to pick it up and heard this voice—a voice I never want to hear again. It said, "darkness rules!" Then there was a smell—not an atmosphere—of evil and I felt I was being dragged down into something. It was like being pushed. I forced myself to wake up. I was sweating like a hog. I looked around my room and thought it was over. Suddenly that pushing sensation started again while I was WIDE AWAKE! Whatever the hell it was (probably was hell), it was pushing me back down to sleep. I don't mean that I felt a bit tired and closed my eyes—it was literally shoving me asleep.[43]

I have left this common REM parasomnia for last as sleep paralysis is comparatively not as well understood as the other forms of weirdness in the night. Like I thought when I was a teen, the experience feels real, not like a dream.

What is sleep paralysis? The primary experience includes feelings of oppression or being held down, as if a weight or force is pushing against the chest, limbs, and throat. When attempts to move are made, the oppression only becomes more forceful. This is accompanied by tremendous feelings of fear and anxiety in the dreamer. Strange bodily misperceptions known as *hypnagogic hallucinations* can occur with sleep paralysis, such as feeling tingly sensations, gravitational shifts, and even realistic out-of-body experiences. Personally, I prefer the term *visions* as it lends a more respectful tone to the experience, whereas "hallucinations" denotes a lack of meaning. Many sleep paralysis experiences also include uncanny perceptions that are literally the stuff of horror movies and ghost stories, such as hearing footsteps approach the bed.

More than half of sleep paralysis nightmares include the distinct awareness of an unknown "sensed presence" in the bedroom.[44] The sensed presence generally is assumed or interpreted to be a horrific monster, otherworldly figure, or ghostly apparition. Anthropologist Shelly Adler terms this unseen entity, in all its cross-cultural forms and variations, as the *nocturnal pressing spirit*.[45] In a minority of cases, the dream hallucinations also reveal the identity apparition or shadowy figure; cultural interpretations vary from demons to old hags, to dangerous spirits or ancestors. The seen entity can be incorporated into the feelings of oppression as a malevolent choking spirit. Seen or unseen, after a few moments the vision dissipates and the muscular paralysis lifts, leaving the sleeper wide awake, in severe emotional distress and certain that the experience was "not a dream."

Sleep paralysis occurs when waking up or falling into sleep. This chapter focuses on recurrent isolated sleep paralysis, which is now considered a variant of nightmare disorder.[46] In its recurrent isolated form, sleep paralysis lasts a few minutes or less, but as a symptom of narcolepsy and sleep apnea, the event can last much longer. Frequent, recurrent episodes throughout the night can be disruptive to daily life and are treated clinically.

To be sure, the sleep paralysis night-mare is one of the most frightening and disturbing experiences that can happen to us, no matter how old we are. The sleep paralysis *night-mare*—the use of the hyphen is to distinguish it from the more "ordinary" REM nightmare—can be brutal in content and emotional tone, especially for children who have had no cultural preparation for the experience. Note that sexual molestation hallucinations during sleep paralysis, known classically as *supernatural assault*, are reported in a minority of cases as well, and are most likely correlated with past trauma, PTSD, as well as anxiety disorders.

Interpreting and Working with Sleep Paralysis Visions

Despite its supernatural scent, awareness during sleep paralysis is well understood as a hiccup in sleep staging known as REM intrusion into wakefulness. Clinical and neurological studies on sleep paralysis have shown that the primary experience of paralysis is REM *muscle atonia*, which our bodies undergo every time we enter REM sleep in order to prevent us from acting out our dreams.[47] When REM intrudes into Stage N1 sleep, that hard to pin down threshold between sleep and wakefulness that often feels like deep relaxation, the dreamer becomes aware of the sudden motor inhibition of skeletal muscles, including the diaphragm. Attempts to gulp in air or gasp in surprise are experienced as resistance focused on the chest and throat; attempts to move feel like an active force is holding the dreamer down.

Around 15–18 percent of the general population has experienced isolated sleep paralysis.[48] Certain groups, including students and psychiatric patients, have higher incidence rates, most likely because these groups are also prone to more sleep disturbances than the general public. Sleep paralysis also has a moderate genetic influence.[49] More importantly, isolated sleep paralysis is considered to be overwhelmingly triggered by factors related to disturbed sleep, similar to night terrors and sleepwalking.

Unfortunately, the hallucinatory aspects of sleep paralysis visions are not as well explained; consequently, parents and caregivers are likely to also be unduly alarmed due to the shockingly realistic feel of these experiences, which are essentially spontaneous altered states of consciousness. Most people, teens especially, are not prepared for waking visions as Western culture does not promote or attend to this class of experience, leading to a rift between observation and beliefs that are passed down through the family and culture as a whole. David Hufford, the medical anthropologist who pioneered the modern revival of sleep paralysis studies in the 1980s, more recently suggested that sleep paralysis should be seen as an *extraordinary spiritual experience*, along with other powerful encounters such as visitation dreams of the dead and out-of-body experiences, all of which are associated with REM intrusion into wakefulness.[50]

Hence, when I was 14 and had my first sleep paralysis nightmare—held down by an evil unseen force while awake and aware—I assumed I was being attacked by a demon. Without a scientific framework, I pulled from a default Christian worldview even though I was raised more as a humanist than anything else. I quickly learned that no one believed or wanted to hear about my experience, and I did not mention it again for over a decade until reading about sleep paralysis in the dream studies literature. As medical anthropologist Shelly Adler discovered while working with Hmong refugees in the United States who suffered collectively from sleep paralysis visions when converting from their traditional beliefs to Christianity, a rift in spiritual beliefs can provide an existential "opening" for the kind of deep anxiety and dread that is correlated with sleep paralysis events.[51] Echoing our analysis of the lingering effects of night terrors and nightmares, I suggest that parents take seriously their adolescents' fear and anxiety when they have awoken from a sleep paralysis night-mare.

In Conclusion

In the simplest terms, when it comes to preventing and managing parasomnias, how can we help our children feel safe and protected in the darkness of the night? Zooming out, how can we build communities that respect the need for rest and relaxation? Antonio Zadra, professor of psychiatry at

Université de Montreal, told me, "Way too many children go to bed too late for their age and are, in effect, chronically sleep deprived."[52] How can we, as parents and caregivers, mirror this protected environment as we redefine our own relationship to *night consciousness*, including the shadowy aspects of life that tug for attention at the periphery of our vision? Rubin Naiman suggests, "The integration of sleep science with personal meaning and spiritual perspectives opens the way to a more expansive, magnificent, and mythic vision of night, a vision that will both clarify the central challenge of our fear of darkness and simultaneously map our journey towards its healing."[53]

Let us start by putting away those distraction devices and relaxing into dusk every night, dimming the lights to signal the time to stop taking in information. Let us attend to the natural process of slowing down and reflecting on the day as we prepare for the next. Let us buttress stressful times with healthy and fun time spent in the fresh air, breathing deeply. Let us respect our children's fears as they mirror our own unanswered questions. There is solace in wondering about the unknown, together.

Notes

1. American Academy of Sleep Medicine, "International Classification of Sleep Disorders," 3rd ed. (Darien, IL: American Academy of Sleep Medicine, 2014).

2. Robert Moss, *Active Dreaming* (Novato: New World Books, 2011); K. Bulkeley and P. Bulkley, *Children's Dreams: Understanding the Most Memorable Dreams and Nightmares of Childhood* (Lanham, MD: Rowman & Littlefield Publisher, 2012).

3. National Sleep Foundation, "New Recommended Sleep Times," accessed December 14, 2015, http://sleepfoundation.org/media-center/press-release/national-sleep-foundation-recommends-new-sleep-times.

4. National Sleep Foundation, "Teens and Sleep; National Sleep Foundation Recommends New Sleep Durations," accessed December 14, 2015, https://sleepfoundation.org/sleep-topics/teens-and-sleep.

5. National Sleep Foundation, "Kids Sleep Less with TV or Computer in Their Bedroom," accessed December 14, 2015, http://www.sleepfoundation.org/alert/kids-sleep-less-tv-computer-their-bedroom.

6. National Sleep Foundation, 2011 poll, "Technology in Sleep," accessed December 14, 2015, http://www.sleepfoundation.org/article/sleep-america-polls/2011-communications-technology-use-and-sleep.

7. "Children with TVs in Their Rooms Sleep Less: Study," Reuters (2008), accessed December 14, 2015, http://www.reuters.com/article/us-children-television-idUSSP8206620080903.

8. J. Van den Bulck, "Adolescent Use of Mobile Phones for Calling and for Sending Text Messages after Lights Out: Results from a Prospective Cohort Study with a One-Year Follow-Up," *Sleep* 30, no. 9 (2007): 1220–1223.

9. National Sleep Foundation, "Sleep in America Poll," (2011), accessed December 14, 2015, https://sleepfoundation.org/sleep-polls-data/sleep-in-america -poll/2011-technology-and-sleep.

10. T. Munezawa et al. "The Association between Use of Mobile Phones after Lights Out and Sleep Disturbances among Japanese Adolescents: A Nationwide Cross-Sectional Survey," *Sleep* 34, no. 8 (2011): 1013–1020.

11. American Academy of Sleep Medicine (2015). "CDC Publishes New State-Specific Analysis of Middle and High School Start Times," accessed December 14, 2015, http://www.aasmnet.org/articles.aspx?id=5735.

12. American Academy of Pediatrics (2014), "Let Them Sleep: AAP Recommends Delaying Start Times of Middle and High Schools to Combat Teen Sleep Deprivation," accessed December 14, 2015, http://www.aasmnet.org/articles.aspx? id=5735.

13. Telegraph (October 9, 2014), "Teenagers to Start School at 10am in Oxford University Sleep Experiment," accessed December 14, 2015, http://www .telegraph.co.uk/news/science/science-news/11148930/Teenagers-to-start-school -at-10am-in-Oxford-University-sleep-experiment.html; M. Fischetti, "School Starts Too Early," accessed December 14, 2015. *Scientific American* (September 1, 2014), http://www.scientificamerican.com/article/school-starts-too-early/.

14. N. Santhi et al. "The Spectral Composition of Evening Light and Individual Differences in the Suppression of Melatonin and Delay of Sleep in Humans," *Journal of Pineal Research* 53, no. 1 (2012): 43–59.

15. M. Bonnet and D. Arand, "Clinical Effects of Sleep Fragmentation versus Sleep Deprivation." *Sleep Medicine Review* 7, no. 4 (2003): 297–310.

16. BBC (August 27, 2007). "Junk Sleep Damaging Teen Health," accessed December 14, 2015, http://news.bbc.co.uk/2/hi/health/6962085.stm.

17. R. Naiman, *Healing Night: The Science and Spirit of Sleeping, Dreaming, and Awakening* (Minneapolis: Syren Book Co., 2006), 5. Italics are not original but for emphasis.

18. W. Dement and C. Vaughn, *The Promise of Sleep* (New York: Delacorte Press, 1999), 457.

19. G. Stores, *Sleep Problems in Children and Adolescents* (Cambridge: Cambridge University Press, 2009), 94.

20. A. Zadra and M. Pilon, "NREM Parasomnias," in *Handbook in Clinical Neurology*, vol. 99 (3rd series), Sleep Disorders, Part 2, P. Montagna and S. Chokroverty, eds. (Amsterdam: Elsevier, 2011), 858.

21. Dement and Vaughn, *The Promise of Sleep*, 211.

22. National Sleep Foundation, "Sleepwalking," accessed December 14, 2015, http://sleepfoundation.org/sleep-disorders-problems/abnormal-sleep-behaviors/ sleepwalking.

23. Zadra and Pilon, *Handbook in Clinical Neurology*, 858.

24. D. Petit et al. "Childhood Sleepwalking and Sleep Terrors: A Longitudinal Study of Prevalence and Familiar Aggregation," *JAMA Pediatrics* (May 4, 2015), doi:10.1001/jamapediatrics.2015.127.

25. Personal communication (9/8/2015).

26. C. Guilleminault et al. "Sleepwalking and Sleep Terrors in Prepubertal Children: What Triggers Them?" *Pediatrics* 111, no. 5 (2003): 17–25, accessed December 14, 2015, http://www.ncbi.nlm.nih.gov/pubmed/12509590.

27. Stores, *Sleep Problems*, 94.

28. Jeremy Taylor, "Sleep Walking, Sleep Talking and Night Terrors," *JeremyTaylor.com* (2007), accessed December 14, 2015, http://www.jeremytaylor.com/dream_work/sleep_walking_sleep_talking_and_night_terrors/index.html.

29. D. Hartman et al. "Is There a Dissociative Process in Sleepwalking and Night Terrors?" *Postgraduate Medical Journal* 77, 2001: 244–249, accessed December 14, 2015, http://pmj.bmj.com/content/77/906/244.full.

30. D. Bates and C. Ellicot, "Teenager Plunges 25ft after Sleepwalking out of her Bedroom Window and Survives without Breaking a Single Bone," *The Daily Mail* (May 19, 2009), accessed December 14, 2015, http://www.dailymail.co.uk/news/article-1184565/Teenager-plunges-25ft-sleepwalking-bedroom-window—survives-breaking-single-bone.html.

31. J. Crone, "Four-Year-Old Norway Girl Sleepwalks 4km," *The Local* (September 15, 2014), Accessed December 14, 2015, http://www.thelocal.no/20140915/three-year-old-girl-sleepwalks-four-km.

32. B. Chang, J. Dusek, and H. Benson, "Psychobiological Changes from Relaxation Response Elicitation: Long-Term Practitioners vs. Novices," *Psychosomatics* 52, no. 6 (2011): 550–559, accessed December 14, 2015, http://dx.doi.org/10.1016/j.psym.2011.05.001.

33. Naiman, *Healing Night*, 48.

34. J. Montplaisir et al. "Parasomnias," in Sudhansu Chokroverty (ed.) *Sleep Disorders Medicine, 4th Edition* (in press). Boston: Butterworth-Heinemann.

35. Zadra and Pilon, *Sleep Disorders Medicine*, 856.

36. Petit et al., *JAMA Pediatrics*, e3.

37. Guilleminault et al., *Pediatrics*.

38. Personal communication (September 8, 2015).

39. Taylor, *Dreamwork*.

40. M. Thorpy, and G. Plazzi, *The Parasomnias and Other Sleep-Related Movement Disorders*. (Cambridge: Cambridge University Press, 2010), 155.

41. D. Kaminer, S. Seedat, and D. Stein, "Post-Traumatic Stress Disorder in Children," *World Psychiatry* 4, no. 2 (2005): 121–125.

42. A. Siegel and K. Bulkeley, "Nightmare Remedies: Helping Your Child Tame the Demons of the Night," *Dream Time* (1998), accessed December 14, 2015, http://asdreams.org/magazine/articles/seigel98dreamcatching.htm.

43. Ryan Hurd, *Sleep Paralysis: A Guide to Hypnagogic Visions and Visitors of the Night* (San Mateo: Hyena Press, 2011), iv.

44. J. Cheyne, "The Ominous Numinous," *Journal of Consciousness Studies* 8, no. 5 & 7 (2001): 133; J. Montplaisir, et al., *Sleep Disorders Medicine*, section "Sleep paralysis."

45. S. Adler, *Sleep Paralysis: Night-mares, Nocebos, and the Mind-Body Connection* (New Brunswick: Rutgers University Press, 2011).

46. J. Montplaisir et al., *Sleep Disorders Medicine*, section "Recurrent Isolated Sleep Paralysis," DSM-V, American Psychological Association.

47. T. Takeuchi et al. "Factors Related to the Occurrence of Isolated Sleep Paralysis Elicited during a Multi-Phase Sleep-Wake Schedule," *Sleep* 25, no. 1 (2002): 89–96.

48. B. Sharpless and J. Barber, "Lifetime Prevalence Rates of Sleep Paralysis: A Systemic Review," *Sleep Medicine Review* 15, no. 5 (2011): 311–315.

49. D. Denis et al. "A Twin and Molecular Genetics Study of Sleep Paralysis and Associated Factors," *Journal of Sleep Research* 24 (2015): 438–446.

50. D. Hufford, "Sleep Paralysis as Spiritual Experience," *Transcultural Psychiatry* 42, no. 1 (2005): 46–77; D. Hufford, "Visionary Spiritual Experiences in an Enchanted World," *Anthropology and Humanism* 35, no. 2 (2010): 142–158.

51. Adler, *Sleep paralysis*, 106–109.

52. Personal communication (August 17, 2015).

53. Naiman, *Healing Night*, 6.

Bibliography

Adler, S. *Sleep Paralysis: Night-mares, Nocebos, and the Mind-Body Connection.* New Brunswick: Rutgers University Press, 2011.

Bates, D. and C. Ellicot. "Teenager Plunges 25ft after Sleepwalking Out of Her Bedroom Window . . . and Survives without Breaking a Single Bone." *The Daily Mail* (May 19, 2009). http://www.dailymail.co.uk/news/article-1184565/Teenager-plunges-25ft-sleepwalking-bedroom-window—survives-breaking-single-bone.html. Accessed December 14, 2015.

Bonnet, M. and D. Arand. "Clinical Effects of Sleep Fragmentation versus Sleep Deprivation." *Sleep Medicine Review* 7, no. 4 (2003): 297–310.

Bulkeley, K. and P. Bulkley. *Children's Dreams: Understanding the Most Memorable Dreams and Nightmares of Childhood.* Lanham, MD: Rowman & Littlefield Publisher, 2012.

"CDC publishes new state-specific analysis of middle and high school start times." *American Academy of Sleep Medicine.* Accessed December 14, 2015. http://www.aasmnet.org/articles.aspx?id=5735.

Chang, B., J. Dusek, and H. Benson. "Psychobiological Changes from Relaxation Response Elicitation: Long-Term Practitioners vs. Novices." *Psychosomatics* 52, no. 6 (2011): 550–559. Accessed December 14, 2015. http://dx.doi.org/10.1016/j.psym.2011.05.001.

Cheyne, J. "The Ominous Numinous." *Journal of Consciousness Studies* 8, no. 5 & 7 (2001): 133–150.

"Children With TVs in Their Rooms Sleep Less: Study." *Reuters*, September 3, 2008. Accessed December 14, 2015. http://www.reuters.com/article/us-children-television-idUSSP8206620080903.

Crone, J. "Four-Year-Old Norway Girl Sleepwalks 4km." *The Local* (September 15, 2014). Accessed December 14, 2015. http://www.thelocal.no/20140915/three-year-old-girl-sleepwalks-four-km.

Dement, W. and C. Vaughn. *The Promise of Sleep*. New York: Delacorte Press, 1999.

Denis, D., C. French, R. Rowe, H. Zavos, P. Nolan, M. Parsons, and A. Gregory. "A Twin and Molecular Genetics Study of Sleep Paralysis and Associated Factors." *Journal of Sleep Research* 24 (2015): 438–446.

Fischetti, M. "School Starts Too Early." *Scientific American*, September 1, 2014. http://www.scientificamerican.com/article/school-starts-too-early/.

Guilleminault, C., L. Palombini, R. Pelayo, and R. Chervin. "Sleepwalking and Sleep Terrors in Prepubertal Children: What Triggers Them?" *Pediatrics* 111, no. 5 (2003): e17–25. Accessed December 14, 2015. http://www.ncbi.nlm.nih.gov/pubmed/12509590.

Hartman, D., A. Crisp, P. Sedgwick, and S. Borrow. "Is There a Dissociative Process in Sleepwalking and Night Terrors?" *Postgraduate Medical Journal* 77 (2001): 244–249. Accessed December 14, 2015. http://pmj.bmj.com/content/77/906/244.full.

Hufford, D. "Sleep Paralysis as Spiritual Experience." *Transcultural Psychiatry* 42, no. 1 (2005): 46–77.

Hufford, D. "Visionary Spiritual Experiences in an Enchanted World." *Anthropology and Humanism* 35, no. 2 (2010): 142–158.

Hurd, R. *Sleep Paralysis: A Guide to Hypnagogic Visions and Visitors of the Night*. San Mateo: Hyena Press, 2011.

International Classification of Sleep Disorders, 3rd ed. Darien, IL: American Academy of Sleep Medicine, 2014.

"Junk Sleep Damaging Teen Health." BBC, August 27, 2007. Accessed December 14, 2015. http://news.bbc.co.uk/2/hi/health/6962085.stm.

Kaminer, D., S. Seedat, and D. Stein. "Post-Traumatic Stress Disorder in Children." *World Psychiatry* 4, no. 2 (2005): 121–125.

"Let Them Sleep: AAP Recommends Delaying Start Times of Middle and High Schools to Combat Teen Sleep Deprivation." *American Academy of Pediatrics*. Accessed December 14, 2015. http://www.aasmnet.org/articles.aspx?id=5735.

Montplaisir, J., A. Zadra, T. Nielsen, and D. Petit. "Parasomnias." In *Sleep Disorders Medicine, 4th Edition*, edited by Sudhansu Chokroverty. Boston: Butterworth-Heinemann, in press.

Moss, R. *Active Dreaming*. Novato: New World Books, 2011.

Munezawa, T., Y. Kaneita, Y. Osaki, H. Kanda, M. Minowa, K. Suzuki, S. Higuchi, J. Mori, R. Yamamoto, and T. Ohida. "The Association between Use of Mobile Phones after Lights Out and Sleep Disturbances among Japanese Adolescents: A Nationwide Cross-Sectional Survey." *Sleep* 34, no. 8 (2011):1013–1020.

Naiman, R. *Healing Night: The Science and Spirit of Sleeping, Dreaming, and Awakening*. Minneapolis: Syren Book Co., 2006.

National Sleep Foundation. "Kids Sleep Less with TV or Computer in Their Bedroom." Accessed December 14, 2015. http://www.sleepfoundation.org/alert/kids-sleep-less-tv-computer-their-bedroom.

National Sleep Foundation. "New Recommended Sleep Times." Accessed December 14, 2015. http://sleepfoundation.org/media-center/press-release/national-sleep-foundation-recommends-new-sleep-times.

National Sleep Foundation. "Sleep in America Poll, 2011." Accessed December 14, 2015. http://www.sleepfoundation.org/article/sleep-america-polls/2011-communications-technology-use-and-sleep.

National Sleep Foundation. "Sleepwalking." Accessed December 14, 2015. http://sleepfoundation.org/sleep-disorders-problems/abnormal-sleep-behaviors/sleepwalking.

National Sleep Foundation. "Teens and Sleep; National Sleep Foundation Recommends New Sleep Durations." February 2, 2015. Accessed December 14, 2015. https://sleepfoundation.org/sleep-topics/teens-and-sleep.

National Sleep Foundation. "Technology in Sleep, 2011 Poll." Accessed December 14, 2015. https://sleepfoundation.org/sleep-pollsdata/sleep-in-america-poll/2011-technology-and-sleep.

Petit, D., M. Pennesti, J. Paquet, A. Desautels, A. Zadra, F. Vitaro, R. Trembla, M. Boivin, and J. Montplaisir. "Childhood Sleepwalking and Sleep Terrors: A Longitudinal Study of Prevalence and Familiar Aggregation." *JAMA Pediatrics* (May 4, 2015): e4. Accessed December 14, 2015. doi:10.1001/jamapediatrics.2015.127.

Santhi, N., H. Thorne, D. van der Veen, S. Johnsen, S. Mills, V. Hommes, L. Schlangen, S. Archer, and D. Dijk. "The Spectral Composition of Evening Light and Individual Differences in the Suppression of Melatonin and Delay of Sleep in Humans." *Journal of Pineal Research* 53, no. 1 (2012): 43–59.

Sharpless, B. and J. Barber. "Lifetime Prevalence Rates of Sleep Paralysis: A Systemic Review." *Sleep Medicine Review* 15, no. 5 (2011): 311–315.

Siegel, A. and K. Bulkeley. "Nightmare Remedies: Helping Your Child Tame the Demons of the Night." *Dream Time* (1998). Accessed December 14, 2015. http://asdreams.org/magazine/articles/seigel98dreamcatching.htm.

Stores, G. *Sleep Problems in Children and Adolescents.* Cambridge: Cambridge University Press, 2009.

Takeuchi, T., K. Fukuda, Y. Sasaki, M. Inugami, and T. Murphy. "Factors Related to the Occurrence of Isolated Sleep Paralysis Elicited during a Multi-Phase Sleep-Wake Schedule." *Sleep* 25, no. 1 (2002): 89–96.

Taylor, J. "Sleep Walking, Sleep Talking and Night Terrors." *JeremyTaylor.com* (2007). Accessed December 14, 2015. http://www.jeremytaylor.com/dream_work/sleep_walking_sleep_talking_and_night_terrors/index.html.

"Teenagers to Start School at 10am in Oxford University Sleep Experiment." *Telegraph*, October 9, 2014. Accessed December 14, 2015. http://www.telegraph.co.uk/news/science/science-news/11148930/Teenagers-to-startschool-at-10am-in-Oxford-University-sleep-experiment.html.

Thorpy, M. and G. Plazzi. *The Parasomnias and Other Sleep-Related Movement Disorders*. Cambridge: Cambridge University Press, 2010.

Van den Bulck, J. "Adolescent Use of Mobile Phones for Calling and for Sending Text Messages after Lights Out: Results from a Prospective Cohort Study with a One-Year Follow-Up." *Sleep* 30, no. 9 (September 1, 2007): 1220–1223.

Zadra, A. and M. Pibon. "NREM Parasomnias." In *Handbook in Clinical Neurology*, vol. 99 (3rd series), Sleep Disorders, Part 2, edited by P. Montagna and S. Chokroverty, 851–868. Amsterdam: Elsevier, 2011.

CHAPTER ELEVEN

War and Peace: Dreaming a Peaceful World into Being

Jean M. Campbell

I am planting some flowers and small trees, making my own garden with great effort. But the war came and I had to leave my house with my family. After that, returning, I found that my garden had been completely destroyed. I didn't give up. I started to plant and make my garden again.

Dameya, age 12

The World at War

On World Refugee Day in 2014, the United Nations High Commission for Refugees (UNHCR) reported that the number of refugees, asylum seekers and internally displaced persons worldwide had, for the first time since the post–World War II era, exceeded 50 million people. The number continues to grow. Although the five top war-affected countries continue to be Afghanistan, Somalia, Iraq, Syria, and Sudan many other countries are suffering from war as well.

According to the UNHCR, "Children below age 18 make up 46 percent of all refugees. In addition, a record 21,300 asylum applications submitted during 2012 were from children who were unaccompanied or separated from their parents. This is the highest number of unaccompanied or separated children that the UNHCR has recorded."[1]

Despite these heartbreaking figures, the number of refugee children treated for post-traumatic stress (PTS) or other psychosocial effects of war on civilian populations, remains negligible.

In their 2003 article concerning the effects of war trauma on adolescents in Angola, published in the groundbreaking book *The Psychological Impact of War Trauma on Civilians: An International Perspective*, authors Teresa McIntyre and Margarida Ventura note that:

> In recent conflicts children and adolescents have been largely the forgotten victims of war. In fact researchers had neglected the study of the psychological impact of war stress on children and adolescents until the 1990s, thereby hindering the development of psychological intervention programs, despite evidence indicating that the younger the victim, the greater the risk of psychological impairment.[2]

Creating the Crystal Birds Dream Program

This lack of attention to the traumatic effects of war on children was the environment in which members of the international group the World Dreams Peace Bridge began, in 2004, to create the Crystal Birds Dream Program for the children of Seasons Art School in Baghdad, Iraq. A full history of the development of this program and its subsequent funding by musician Carlos Santana's Milagro Foundation can be found in my 2006 book *Group Dreaming: Dreams to the Tenth Power;*[3] but a brief synopsis of these events follows, along with the rationale for use of the program with war-traumatized children. The program we created is designed to be facilitated by any caring adult ready to listen to children's dreams.

In 2003, in the middle of the largest global antiwar protests ever seen, members of the World Dreams Peace Bridge agreed that they should incubate dreams about what to do for the people whose country was soon to be invaded. In the next few weeks, over 30 members of the online group: people of all ages, from many countries and all walks of life, found themselves dreaming about the children of Iraq. As a group of "dream activists," people who believe that not only do dreams provide personal information but can also be used to guide the actions of individuals and society, what became clear to us was that our dreams were inviting us to become involved with the children of a country at war.

Even as the bombs began falling on Baghdad, members of the Peace Bridge were looking for ways to connect with the children there, to aid them in some way that would soften the terrors of destruction. Through the aid of Kathy Kelly, founder of the organization Voices for Creative Non-violence and a member of the Christian Peacekeeping volunteers who remained in Baghdad as "human shields" after the start of the war there, we were able to connect with Emad Hadi, the director of Seasons Art School in Baghdad. And we began to follow our dreams by providing musical instruments and soft, stuffed toys for the children there.

Seasons Art School was one of the first Nongovernmental Organizations (NGOs) developed in Baghdad. It functioned as a pre-school/after-school program for boys and girls under the age of 14. As we became more acquainted with the program and the people who ran it, we exchanged messages with the children via e-mail, received photos of paintings the children created for the Children's Peace Train (another project of the World Dreams Peace Bridge, developed in 2001), and determined that we should create a program that could be used by this community to aid the children in understanding the dreams and nightmares they were almost certainly having.

Because the World Dreams Peace Bridge was primarily focused on dreams submitted to the group by its members rather than any sort of academic credentials, it was not clear until we began to create the Crystal Birds Dream Program, what an extraordinary group of people we had pulled together, and how remarkably capable they might be in the creation of a dream program for war-traumatized children. With the support of other members of the group, four people from the Peace Bridge became involved in developing the program: Dr. May Tung of San Francisco, California, formerly from Beijing, China; Dr. Brenda Mallon, from Manchester, England; Ilkin Sungu, an internationally known journalist from Istanbul, Turkey; and I.

What we discovered, as we began to work on this program, was that not only had children who suffered the fate of "collateral damage" to civilians in war been a population neglected by researchers; but that there were absolutely no current studies of the effects of war on the dreams of children.

Fortunately for the developing Crystal Birds Dream Program, we found that with the aforementioned group, we had collected a coalition of highly trained experts. May Tung was internationally known for her work in intercultural studies. Having escaped from China during World War II, she was herself an immigrant. As a clinical psychologist in San Francisco, she had directed intercultural training programs for therapists and written books and articles about counseling Chinese Americans. It was May Tung who reiterated to the group that the program we were working on needed to be viable for all traumatized children, no matter what their origin or nationality.

Brenda Mallon, who donated copies of her book *Dream Time with Children: Learning to Dream, Dreaming to Learn* to program facilitators, was born in England to Irish parents. She trained as a teacher and counselor, and in 1980 was one of the first people to introduce counseling into schools in Britain. We found ourselves in total agreement with the opening lines of

Dream Time with Children which say: "Children need to dream because dreaming is part of the cognitive process where learning is laid down and memories classified and stored. Anyone who cares about their child's progress, emotionally and academically, needs to understand the powerful influence of dreams."[4]

Ilkin Sungu, part of an affluent and influential family in Turkey, had twin sons in college at the time of the war in Iraq. Thus she particularly identified with the plight of both the students and staff of Seasons Art School. It was Ilkin, a strong telepathic and precognitive dreamer, who took the lead in fund-raising and collecting materials in support of the nascent dream program.

We were fortunate to have, from Baghdad, another active supporter of the plan to create the Crystal Birds Dream Program. In addition to school director, Emad Hadi, a graduate student in arts and theater at the University of Baghdad, we received the assistance of Dr. Ali Rashed. Dr. Ali, a child psychotherapist, was the person who tested and looked after the children at Seasons Art School. His area of expertise was post-traumatic stress. As he told us: "I have been caring for traumatized children since before this war began. Iraq has been at war throughout the lifetimes of most of the children here, and many of the adults." Through Ali and his colleagues, we not only met, via the Internet, many of the people in Iraq who were working with children, but learned a great deal about how childhood trauma was treated there.

Foundational Concepts for the Crystal Birds Dream Program

Because of the interest in creating a dream program for children shown by all of the adults involved, there was no doubt that we were going to develop a dream program; but to our delight, as soon as we began talking about this possible program, the children of Seasons Art School took matters into their own hands. A group of 20 young people at the school, children between the ages of 10 and 14, both boys and girls, spontaneously self-selected to work with their dreams. By the end of 2004, these children had created a name for themselves: The Crystal Birds. They found a classroom, which they decorated. And they were ready to dream themselves into a brighter future.

Those of us involved with creating the program began to look at some foundational concepts for working with the dreams of traumatized children. We agreed that, whether the trauma derived from war, or from violence of any other kind: (1) Children need the encouragement of adults to both dream and believe in the importance of their dreams. (2) No matter the culture or ethnic group from which the child comes, or from where the trauma originates, children can be taught to receive guidance and assistance from their dreams. (3) Because a primary tenet of working with trauma is that the traumatized individual needs a "safe space" in which to work with the trauma, the program must contain ways to establish that safe space. (4) The dream belongs to the dreamer. Children have an innate sense of the meanings of their dreams. Rather than interpreting dreams for children, it is important that others (including other children) listen attentively and respect the dreamer's innate understanding of meaning. (5) Finally, it is essential to avoid generalizations about dream meanings, even though many children come from cultures in which meaning may be ascribed to certain symbols in dreams.

This last point we found to be particularly important, in light of research that has been conducted on dreams among adult survivors of war trauma, and even among those who may instigate the violence. It is so very easy, in a research environment, to make generalizations about cultures but like any generalizations, these need to be examined. For example, researchers Deirdre Barrett and Jaffar Behbehani, in their study of post-traumatic nightmares in Kuwait following the Iraqi invasion, state somewhat categorically: "Muslim and Arab folk beliefs about dreams focus so exclusively on using them to foretell the future that few assumptions are made (such as those taken as a given by Western traditions) of dream content arising from the dreamer's past."[5] Though it is true that there is a strong tradition of dreams being used to foretell the future in Arab cultures, it is important to not prejudge. We discovered that the children from whom we collected dreams had a wide variety of both dreams and interpretations of them.

It is also important for us to look at the context of research done on Islamic cultures today, since considerable research has been done (and continues to be conducted) on the dreams of Islamic terrorists. For example, researcher Iain Ross Edgar, who follows the news reports of dreams among Islamic terrorists, says in his 2015 article "Dreams of Islamic State" in the online journal *Perspectives on Terrorism*: "The Islamic tradition distinguishes between three types of dreams: the true dream (*al-ru'ya*), the false dream, which may come from the devil, and the meaningless everyday dream (*hulm*)."[6]

Although certainly some children, growing up in any culture, will take on the beliefs about dreams that adults propound, the essential fact is that the dreams of war-traumatized children are much more in line with what Cole P. Dodge wrote in 1992 about the dreams of children in war situations in Sudan, Uganda, and Mozambique:

Children may be reluctant to go to sleep for fear of dreams or nightmares. They may demand company until they fall asleep, they may want to sleep together with others, or desire to have a light or fire. Even adolescents can react that way. Most children will have dreams related to what they experienced following traumatic events. . . . Traumatic dreams bring little relief, but when they are talked about and the child is given some understanding of why such dreams occur, this can help in preventing them. As children are able to put their feelings into words, night terrors tend to disappear.[7]

An Eight-Week Program for Working with Dreams

What follows is a condensed version of the Crystal Birds Dream Program created for the children of Baghdad. The original program, as funded by the Milagro Foundation, was designed to extend over an eight-week period, providing three sessions of one- or two-hour duration per week.

Week One: How to Remember Your Dreams

1. Go to bed as soon as you feel sleepy. You remember your dreams best when you get a good night's sleep.
2. Just before going to bed, say to yourself (out loud or in your head): "Tonight I will have wonderful dreams. When I wake up in the morning, I will remember my dreams."
3. Keep your dream journal, with a pencil or pen, by the side of your bed. Every morning make a record of the dreams you had the night before. You might want to use a copy of the Dream Report handout.
4. When you wake up in the morning, stay in bed for a little while to write and remember your dreams. If you jump right out of bed, you may not remember your dreams clearly. Before getting out of bed, take a few minutes and write down your dreams; or if you like, draw a picture in your journal about what happened in the dream.
5. Sharing a dream with another person soon after the dream is another way to remember a dream.

As mentioned earlier, several dream report forms are provided during week one of the program. These dream reports include questions on such topics as: "A Recent Dream," "My Favorite Dream," and "My Favorite Nightmare." In each case, the individual is asked to give the name, date, and description of the dream. Children are also asked to state how they felt when they had the dream, and to circle the emotions that apply: happy, angry, curious, afraid, joyful, worried, excited, peaceful, sad, anxious, and so on. They are asked to describe the characters (people, animals, and others) in the dream; note where the dream takes place, and also to draw a picture of the dream. These first dream reports are essential, in order for the adults facilitating the program to get an idea of the dreamer's state of mind. Sometimes it can become evident that the child needs deeper and more individualized work than a dream group can provide.

Week one of the program also provides a list of some of the types of dreams people have, and describes them: adventure dreams, learning dreams, lucid dreams, magical dreams, nightmares, practice dreams, problem-solving dreams, vacation dreams, and shared dreams. Some questions are posed for children to think about and discuss: When you say, "I had a dream," what do you mean? What happens when you dream? Where do you go when you dream? What happens to your physical body when you dream? What do you think your "dream body" is made out of? What is the value of dreaming?

Week Two: A Safe Space/A Happy Place

The objective for the week is to provide the idea that, even in the worst situations, we can find inner strength and accomplish a lot. In order to be safe and happy, people need a place that is safe and comfortable. That place can be found both in waking locations and in dreams.

Week two introduces the topic of dream incubation. The instructions are given: "For two days before you dream, tell yourself, 'I can dream whatever I want.' On the third day, before falling asleep tell yourself, 'Tonight I will dream about _____,' and then see what happens."

Also some "rules of the game" are laid down for when the group begins a discussion of dreams. They involve listening: When we talk about dreams in a group, listening is very important. Let the dreamer tell the dream, all the way through, without interruption. Try to listen with respect. Pretend it is your own dream you are hearing. Talk only when you want to. Dreams are very private and special. Do not let anyone else tell you when to talk about a dream or tell you what your dream means. Do not tell. Do not talk about someone else's dreams or tell what someone talked about to anyone outside the group unless you have the permission of the person who said it. Be kind, fair, and sensitive to others in your dream group.

The primary exercise of week two is to create a shadow box. Necessary materials for this are small, empty boxes, magazine pictures and small objects like toy animals, stones, and twigs. Glue, paint, and other art supplies may be needed as well. For this exercise, children are told that they will use the shadow boxes to create their safe place. They can write a description first, or draw a picture of what their safe space/happy place might look like, and then use the shadow boxes to create a three-dimensional model. At the end of this session, children are given the suggestion to incubate a dream about their own safe space. In the final session of the week, children can discuss the answers to questions such as: Did you dream of a safe, happy space? (For some, this exercise will bring the onset of feelings that there is no such place, and this question needs to be addressed.) What did your space look like? What did you like best about it? If you did not dream about a safe space, why do you think that happened?

Only about half of the people who try this exercise find a safe and happy place on their first attempt to dream it. Tell children that they can keep trying. We can exercise our dreaming self just the way we exercise our bodies when we are awake.

Week Three: What Does My Dream Mean?

Session one of this week asks children to stand in a circle. Then they are asked to notice how they stand. "Do you stand with your back straight, or do you slump?" "Do you stand more on one leg or another?" "If someone were to describe what you look like when you stand, how do you think they would describe you?"

Then, still in a circle, we suggest that the children select a dream. This does not have to be a recent dream, but can be a dream that has been important from any time in the past. Then they are asked to select a character from the dream (an animal, an object, or a person who stands out). "Without talking," children are instructed, "take one step to the right in the circle. Step into your dream character. Become the character from your dream. Notice how you stand. Feel that. If your dream character stands or moves in a certain way, do that."

Then they are asked to take a step to the left. "Step back into your waking self. How do you feel? How do you stand? We may feel differently in our dreams from how we feel when we are awake. Each character in our dreams, each object, is part of our self too, with something to teach us."

Questions to think about and discuss with this exercise include: How did I feel as myself? As my dream character? What did my dream character tell me about itself? What did I learn about myself?

A second exercise for this week involves what is known as *gestalt* work. Choose a partner in the group. Each one of the partners selects a dream to tell. As the dreams are told, the partner listens attentively to the other person's dream. Then a particular character (animal, object) from the dream is selected by the dreamer. The partner asks the following questions:

Who are you? Could you describe yourself? Why are you here in this dream? What do you have to offer (the dreamer)? What do you need? What can (the dreamer) do for you? Make sure to write down the answers to these questions. At the end of the exercise, students are asked to return to the circle, allowing anyone who wants or needs to talk about what happened to do so.

The final session of week three is a discussion of symbols. That is, in dreams one thing may stand for another. For example, sometimes people will symbolize a new project or new idea in life by dreaming about a garden where things are growing or dream of other things that indicate a new beginning. In a dream, you are not just yourself, but the other characters too. If we dream something again and again, the dream probably contains an important symbol, with an important message. Here are some suggestions that can be used. What is your symbol for wealth or riches in your dreams? (Draw it.) What is your symbol for happiness in your dreams? (Draw it.) What is your symbol for fear in your dreams? (Draw it.) What is your symbol for safety in your dreams? (Draw it.) What is your symbol for pride and self-respect in your dreams? (Draw it.) Discussion about the drawings can be held after each of the drawings is done, or can be held at the end of the session.

Week Four: Being Awake in the Dream

Week four begins with a question: "Has anyone in the group ever had a dream where you knew you were dreaming even though you were still in the dream?" If some people answer yes, let those people tell the dreams they had. Ask this question next: "And then what did you do?" There are people who have these types of dreams, called lucid dreams, quite often.

Here is an exercise for the whole week: See if you can become awake in your dreams. Can you recognize that the dream is happening while you are dreaming? What happens if you say to yourself or others in the dream: "I'm dreaming?" What can you do in this kind of dream that you don't do in other dreams? Let's have an adventure.

Exercise: Pick a dream adventure you have had. In groups of three, tell your partners your dream. See if you can act out your dream, letting your partners play the roles of other people or objects in your dream. You can tell your partners exactly what you want them to say or do. This exercise will probably need to be carried over to the third session of the week, because it may take some time to stage the dreams.

Now children are instructed, "With your partners from the last session, act out the high point of your adventure dream in front of the group.

Your partners will be your supporting cast. This time, rather than using words, you are going to use as few words as possible, no words at all if you can do it. This is called dream pantomime. Be sure to pick only the most important part of your dream, the part you think of as most important, to pantomime in front of the group. How does this feel? What did you learn about yourself from your dream? You can answer these questions in the group, or write them down in your dream journal."

Week Five: Who Dreams?

In the first session of the week, ask the group: Did anyone have a dream recently they would like to tell the group? (Note: this question can be repeated as often as time allows, or if there are many dreams, the group can pick one or two dreams they would most like to work with.)

"Today, we are going to work with adopting a dream."

In this exercise, once the group has listened to a dream, each person in the group spends some time thinking about what this dream might mean if the dream had occurred to him or her rather than the original dreamer. Tell students: "Some people believe that your dream could have meaning to me too, if I would only listen to it carefully and 'pretend' the dream is mine. In other words, we can 'adopt' another person's dream as our own, in order to explore what it might mean." In the ensuing discussion, statements made about the dream need to begin with: "If that were my dream ..." and be completed with a statement of what the dream might mean if it were dreamed by the speaker. Make sure that dreams are told slowly, clearly, and in the present tense. Be patient with this process. Sometimes when we listen to a dream, it is almost as if we fall into the dream ourselves.

At the end of this week's first session, give the children the following assignment for the week. "Do other people you know have dreams? Who dreams? Talk with some of the people you know and ask them the following questions: Do you remember your dreams? Do you enjoy your dreams? What have you learned from your dreams? What do you think is the reason people dream? Write down the answers you hear."

An important note for faculty: All of us have emotions that are unexpressed. Sometimes we encounter these emotions while working with a dream, because dreams do not hold back. They let us know exactly how we are feeling. The way that a teacher or group facilitator deals with emotions is important. If we take the attitude that expressing certain emotions, even in a dream, is bad, then what we are teaching a child is that some emotions are bad. Instead, we can teach children that emotions themselves are neither bad nor good, but how we act on our feelings can be either healing or harmful to ourselves and others. If feelings come up in the context of the group, you may want to allow the dreamer to express the feelings in some way. A person who is angry can hit or yell at a soft pillow. A person who is sad can express the feelings with tears. Especially for children, having someone willing to listen, really listen, can be the most important of all.

Take some time in the group for people to talk about what they learned from asking other people questions about dreaming. Ask students to write an essay (an in-class essay) that answers these questions: "What do I believe is true about dreams? Is that the same answer or a different one from that given by someone I talked with about dreams?" In the discussion that follows, ask students if they can answer these questions as well: "In my area of the world, what do people seem to believe about dreams? Historically, in my family or the world, what are the different beliefs people seem to have about dreams? Are these beliefs about dreams true all over the world? What do I believe about dreams?"

Week Six: Do Dreams Ever Come True?

Building on weeks one, two, and four, the exercises for this week will be about long-term creativity. As needed, provide information about precognitive dreaming.

Exercise: Draw a Dream.

Students are told to pick a dream that they would like to draw. In making this picture, they are to use only the middle of the paper. Once the dream picture is complete, each person in the group can say a few words about his or her picture and the dream it represents. This exercise, however, is about what is "outside the dream." Once the dreams are described the facilitator then asks the following questions (or types of questions), giving time for participants to add to the dream in the middle of the paper: What is happening on the other side of the wall? (Draw it.) What is on the other side of the hill? (Draw it.) What is behind the chair? (Draw it.) What is in the next room? (Draw it.) Take some time discussing what has been drawn, and what it might tell the dreamer about the message of the dream.

Exercise for the week: "Pick someone (preferably someone from the group) and see if the two of you can share a dream." What does dream sharing mean in this context? Sometimes people actually dream the same dream on the same night, or their dreams contain very similar elements. And sometimes, if the dreamers are lucid dreaming, they might even know they are sharing while the dream goes on. Tell students: "Before you go to sleep on the night you are planning to dream with someone, say to yourself: 'I can dream about my dream partner, and remember my dream.' "

When the next group session begins, ask students to sit in a circle, allowing each person to briefly tell a dream that has been dreamed since the last group meeting. Then compare the dreams. Were there things that were alike in the dreams? Did anyone dream a member of the group? Did anyone in the group share a dream with his or her dream partner? Did anyone have a dream very similar to someone else in the group?

Ask students to share a story created from a dream. Divide the group into groups of four. Ask each person to choose a character from a dream, someone or something important to the dream, and to write a description of that character. Then students are asked to begin to write a story about this character. At the end of 10 minutes, no matter what is happening in the story, students are asked to pass the story to the person seated on the dreamer's right. The next person continues the story. This process continues until the original story returns to the dreamer. Ask students: "What happened to your dream character? How do you feel about it?" Allow time for discussion.

Week Seven: Can I Use My Dreams to Solve a Problem?

At the beginning of this week, a list of people who have used dreams to solve problems is presented to the group. For example, singer/songwriter John Lennon, well known as one of the Beatles, often dreamed songs he would later turn into hits. The same is true for British musician, Sting. Author Alice Walker, who calls herself "author and medium" often dreams "the ancestors" or people who are characters in her books. Similarly, author Robert Louis Stevenson told people that his "brownies" came to him while he was asleep with pieces of the stories he would later write. Inventor Eli Whitney created the cotton gin after having a dream about it, and physicist Niels Bohr solved a major problem in nuclear physics in his dreams.

Exercise for the week: "Pick a problem in your life you would like to solve. See if you can incubate a dream this week that gives you the information necessary to solve the problem."

Ask students: "Have you ever had a scary dream? What can you do to solve the problem of being scared in a dream or scared by the dream?" Break the group into two smaller groups, each with a leader or facilitator. Then ask who wants to tell a scary dream? Let the dreamer stand in the middle of the circle to tell the dream. The dreamer can even act out the dream as it is being told. What suggestions do other members of the group have for the person in the dream? What are some things that could be done in the dream to make it feel less scary? The dreamer can act out the suggestions too.

Then tell group members to think about the problem they have selected for this week's exercise. Ask them to write a story or a poem, or make a picture or set of pictures, describing the problem and what can be done to solve it. Ask students to share the results with the rest of the group, and discuss the solutions.

Week Eight: Honoring the Dream

This week, the final week of the group, we ask students to pick a dream they have had that feels extremely important. It could be a dream from last night, or it might be a dream from long ago. Tell them: "This week, you are going to honor that dream by creating something that represents the dream in waking life. It might be a drawing or a story. It might be a wood carving, or something made of fabric. Whatever it is, you might ask your dreaming self what object you can create that will honor this dream the most." The week concludes with the following Dream Honoring Ceremony:

With faculty joining the students, stand or sit on the floor in a circle. Ask students to first tell the dream that will be honored, telling it slowly, as if it was happening right now. Following the dream telling, the dreamer is asked to show his or her "dream honor object" to the group. If this is a story or a poem, the dreamer can be asked to read part or all of it. Then the "dream honor object" is placed in the middle of the circle.

After everyone has finished this part of the exercise, ask people to close their eyes for the following instructions: "Say thank you to your dreams. Say thank you to your dreaming self for providing the dreams. And silently thank whoever or whatever you believe contributes to your dreams. If this group has been fun for you, or a help for you, then keep writing your dreams in a daily journal, and share your dreams with other people you know. If we continue to exercise our dreaming muscles, our dreams will continue to grow and to help us grow."

Week Nine: Or Before the Final Goodbye is Said

Repeat the evaluation forms from Week One. This may take some time, but students can answer the following questions: "Has anything changed with your dreams since this group began?" Ask them to write a paragraph or two about these changes.

Children's Dreams

As soon as it became clear that we would receive funding for the Crystal Birds Dream Program, those involved with creating the program began to collect the dreams of children from Seasons Art School and from work-shops sponsored by the Department of Education in Baghdad. Clearly, "Shock and Awe," the massive bombing of Baghdad, had left its mark.

As reported by his father, Ahmed, age six, had a dream shortly after the war began. This was Ahmed's first recorded dream, possibly the first dream he had ever recalled.

He saw a pigeon come to the window, stopping there. When the window was opened, the pigeon came inside. The pigeon was carrying a toy, like the devil. The pigeon had broken the devil toy with his beak. When Ahmed saw the pigeon come inside, he ran away.

Another child displaced by the bombings, 10-year-old Noor, described the process of looking for a new home in her dream:

We were all searching for a house and we find an old woman (around 45 or 50). This woman had a very big house, and she gave two rooms to me.

Thirteen-year-old Mustafa recorded the only dream which (in terms of Muslim dream tradition discussed earlier in this chapter) might be called a "religious" dream:

In the dream, he says, his family goes to the holy city of Najaf. Mustafa says: *We saw the big sea, and I saw a man with a light. The man had wings. This man opened Amman Ali's grave and Amman Ali woke up from the grave. There was a thief who stole a bag from this man with wings. I got the bag back and returned it to the man with wings.*

Mohammed, age 11, however wrote:

I dreamed I am an engineer. The first work I did on returning to my neighbor-hood was to rebuild my damaged school. I named this school: "The Future School."

In comparison, one might look at the dreams of one of the most famous survivors of war trauma in the world, Malala Yousafzai, a young girl from Pakistan's Swat Valley, known now as the youngest-ever winner of the Nobel Peace Prize. In her book *I am Malala*, coauthored with Christina Lamb, Malala writes: "The first Journal entry in 'The Diary of Gul Makai' for the BBC in January 2009 (written under a pseudonym when Malala was 15) reports a dream under the heading I AM AFRAID!. 'I had a terrible dream last night filled with military helicopters and Taliban.' I have had such dreams since the launch of the military operation in Swat."[8]

After many months of preparation, the Crystal Birds Dream Program ended in Baghdad almost before it had begun. Late in 2005, with unrest deepening in the city, Emad Hadi wrote to us that a friend had been killed, and his own life had been threatened. It was no longer safe for the children to come to school, as even children were being targeted by snipers and stolen off the streets to sell for ransom. Although there were plans to reopen Seasons Art School in another location, this did not happen.

Conclusions

One could say that, in terms of statistical research, there were no results from the Crystal Birds Dream Program. The funded use of this program with the children in Baghdad was too brief, too inconclusive for results to be noted.

Yet in human terms, we might see this program as a success. That a small group of dreamers, the World Dreams Peace Bridge, was led by their dreams to make contact with civilians in a country where, once the invasion began, all civilian mail and other communications stopped, was nothing short of a miracle. Money and toys were sent by us through Jordan, requiring a dangerous road trip from Baghdad. That children in a country being bombed and terrorized were able to see "foreigners" as possible friends rather than enemies was quite amazing. That these children should feel, for whatever small amount of time, that someone was listening to their dreams and listening to their stories, was also considered important by participants. In fact, some of the people involved have continued to communicate with their international friends.

In a world torn by war, there is more need than ever before to pay attention to the dreams of children. In Iraq, as in most countries of the Middle East, over 75 percent of the population is under the age of 25—a population comprised of young adults. In this context, perhaps more than any other, children are the future. The dreams of these children will become the future. The Crystal Birds Dream Program is not only an important step toward listening to the dreams of child survivors of war, but it is also a way toward peace.

Notes

1. United Nations High Commission for Refugees, "New UNHCR Report Says Global Forced Displacement at 18-Year High," *UNHCR News Stories*, June 19, 2013, http://www.unhcr.org/51c071816.html.

2. Teresa M. McIntyre and Margarida Ventura, "Children of War: Psychosocial Sequelae of War Trauma in Angolan Adolescents, in *The Psychological Impact of War Trauma on Civilians*, ed. Stanley Krippner and Teresa McIntyre (Westport, CT: Praeger, 2003), 39.

3. Jean Campbell, *Group Dreaming: Dreams to the Tenth Power* (Norfolk, VA: Donning, 2006), 175–188.

4. Brenda Mallon, *Dream Time with Children* (London: Jessica Kingsley Publishers, 2002), 9.

5. Deirdre Barrett and Jaffar Behbehani, "Post-Traumatic Nightmares in Kuwait Following the Iraqi Invasion," in *The Psychological Impact of War Trauma on Civilians*, ed. Stanley Krippner and Teresa McIntyre (Westport, CT: Praeger, 2003), 139.

6. Iain Ross Edgar, "The Dreams of Islamic State," *Perspectives in Terrorism* 9, no. 4 (2015): 72–84, http://www.terrorismanalysts.com/pt/index.php/pot/article/viewFile/455/903.

7. Cole P. Dodge, *Reaching Children in War: Sudan, Uganda and Mozambique* (London: Jessica Kingsley, 1992), 35–36.

8. Malala Yousafzai with Christina Lamb, *I Am Malala* (New York, London: Back Bay Books, Little Brown and Co., [2013], 2015), 155.

Bibliography

Barrett, Deirdre and Jaffar Behbehani. "Post-Traumatic Nightmares in Kuwait Following the Iraqi Invasion." In *The Psychological Impact of War Trauma on Civilians: An International Perspective*, edited by Stanley Krippner and Teresa McIntyre, 135–142, Westport, CT: Praeger, 2003.

Edgar, Iain R. "The Dreams of Islamic State." *Perspectives in Terrorism* 9, no. 4 (2015): 72–84. http://www.terrorismanalysis.com.

Campbell, Jean. *Group Dreaming: Dreams to the Tenth Power*. Norfolk VA: Wordminder Press, 2006.

Dodge, Cole. *Reaching Children in War: Sudan, Uganda, and Mozambique*. London: Jessica Kingsley Publishers, 1992.

Mallon, Brenda. *Dream Time with Children*. London: Jessica Kingsley Publishers, 2002.

McIntyre, Teresa and Margarida Venturo. "Children of War: Psychosocial Sequelae of War Trauma. In *The Psychological Impact of War Trauma on Civilians: An International Perspective*, edited by Stanley Krippner and Teresa McIntyre, 39–53, Westport, CT: Praeger, 2003.

United Nations High Commission for Refugees. "*New UNHCR Report Says Global Forced Displacement at 18-year High*." Geneva, Switzerland: UNHCR News Stories, June 19, 2013. http://www.unhcr.org/51c071816.html.

Yousafzai, Malala with Christine Lamb. *I am Malala*. New York: Back Bay Books/ Little Brown and Company, 2013.

PART FOUR

Extraordinary Dreams

CHAPTER TWELVE

Young Superheroes of the Dreamtime: Dreams of Time, Space, and the Future

Linda Mastrangelo

The simplest way to visualize a Kerr wormhole is to think of Alice's Looking Glass. Anyone walking through the Looking Glass would be transported instantly into Wonderland, a world where animals talked in riddles and common sense wasn't so common.

Michio Kaku

For a child, the idea of one day becoming an astronaut traveling through space carries with it exciting possibilities, adventures, and explorations. What if we took this notion even farther and suggested that, not unlike Alice who ventures into the rabbit hole, there are children who actually do travel to fantastical worlds . . . in the Dreamtime.

There is even a name ascribed to this role that goes back to our ancient ancestry: the oneironaut or "dream traveler" who dreams of time and space and even the future through "psi" experiences to gain knowledge in order to be of service to the community. *Psi* is a term used to qualify psychic or paranormal dreams that include precognition, telepathy, premonitions, and prophecy. Each carries with it subtle nuances. Precognitive (or "precog") dreams are dreams of an actual event (likely traumatic) that then occurs in waking life. Premonition dreams predict individual futures, while prophetic dreams affect the collective. Psi dreams also include journeying to different realms through a gateway or portal while "lucid" or conscious that one is dreaming. This phenomenon is often referred to as "the wormhole effect" in quantum theory and in indigenous cosmology it is the World Tree or "Axis Mundi."[1]

According to psychologist Carl Jung[2] and many other contemporary researchers in this field,[3] children not only experience these types of extraordinary dreams, but they are quite commonplace.

Tragically, however, in the "dream-deprived" culture of most of the world today, these dreams are often dismissed as folly and children are told "it was just a dream" or "only your imagination." This seemingly harmless rejection of childhood experiences is not unusual and in many cases, these offhanded dismissals can lead to isolation, low self-esteem, mistrust of authority figures and mental health issues.[4]

In this chapter, the role of child as oneironaut and its links to lucid dreams, quantum physics, and indigenous science/cosmology will be introduced along with the confluence of past travelers like inventor Nikola Tesla and Mexican revolutionary Teresa Urrea. My own childhood and lucid dreaming journey will also be shared, as these experiences brought me to my own work and calling as a therapist and researcher specializing in dreams.

Specific case studies of children's psi dreams will also be presented here, as well as psychoeducational tools for parents, educators, and mental health professionals to help identify and explore these phenomenal dreams of time, space, and the future so we can nurture our superheroes of the Dreamtime. For it is the oneironaut, working in conjunction with the physicist, who will open up new realms of possibilities and the great mysteries of our time!

How do we begin?

As a society, we must first share our own dreams; we must share our stories. We must take that leap into the unknown.

Where It All Begins: Childhood in Borderland

By sharing our dreams, we are also sharing the story of the Universe. And as psychologist James Hillman poignantly highlighted in his opus *The Soul's Code: In Search of Character and Calling*, we must first look to childhood as a signal of the Call as "an urge out of nowhere, a fascination, a peculiar turn of events struck like an annunciation: This is what I must do, this is what I've got to have. This is who I am."[5]

Hillman cites the biographies of famous people such as Mahatma Gandhi and Ella Fitzgerald where a pattern of "the Call" or genius emerged in the early stages of life. As children we are much more in tune with our destiny than as adults.[6] Dreams can give us the map to this terrain of who we once were, where we are now, and possible futures. This means that, as the keepers of children's stories and dreams, we can find clues to the Call to help support children in their journeys toward their authentic selves and the superheroes they are destined to become.

Carl Jung, in his autobiography *Memories, Dreams, Reflections* writes of his lifelong struggle with his own destiny and expressing his extraordinary experiences:

> As a child I felt myself to be alone, and I am still, because I know things and must hint at things which others apparently know nothing of, and for the most part do not want to know. Loneliness does not come from having no people about one, but from being unable to communicate the things that seem important to oneself, or from holding certain views which others find inadmissible.[7]

My own rich dream life began in childhood where the veil between the different worlds was quite thin. Coined by the nineteenth-century French psychologist L. F. Alfred Maury, hypnagogia is derived from two Greek words, *hypnos* (sleep) and *agogeus* (guide, or leader). It is that brief transition between wakefulness and sleep and has many names including "borderland state," the "half-dream state," and the "pre-dream condition."[8] My personal experiences in the hypnagogic state have included mandala-like spiral patterns, audio phenomena in the form of harmonic tones, singing and disembodied voices, and even visits from elemental beings and "ghosts" that have passed over.

These occurrences terrified me as a child, and like Jung I had no context or adult guidance to make sense of them. They were amplified when I was eight years old and my family moved into a 100-year-old house. Though I had my own room for the first time, I learned I was not alone. At night, I would see, hear, or feel energies or presences in the room. Other times I experienced a type of "stretching" as if my body was elongating or trying to come out of my body like in an out-of-body experience (OBE).

I discovered years later, through researching my hometown, that there was deep trauma not only tied to the house and a little girl who died there but also tied to the land itself, due to series of massacres between the colonists and indigenous tribes. Perhaps I was picking up on residual energies. Carl Jung remarks on this phenomenon: "The child born in a country takes something of that land, it is the secret influence of the place."[9]

Though this time period in my childhood was extremely isolating, I also have strong memories of benevolent beings in my room watching over me. I felt that all through this frightening process I was being held in some way by wise teachers or what some call "the invisible ones."

The visionary philosopher Rudolph Steiner emphasized the importance of the hypnagogic state where we often have extraordinary visions, perhaps in the form of geometric shapes and patterns of bright light or we might have auditory experiences of loud knocking or familiar voices or, even more dramatically, a supernatural heightening of our senses, visitation dreams and perhaps even more profoundly, answers to life's biggest mysteries.[10] This state is also known for eliciting lucid dreams.

The Marquis d'Hervey de Saint-Denys spoke of "rêves lucides" or "lucid dreams" in his 1867 book *Les Rêves et les Moyens de les Diriger* (Dreams and Ways to Guide Them) as realizing that you are dreaming while in a dream state;[11] or as the American Psychological Association (APA) defines it, a lucid dream is "a dream in which the sleeper is aware that he or she is dreaming and may be able to influence the progress of the dream narrative."[12]

It was clear that my childhood, and lucid dreaming experiences, were pointing to a calling; I was here to help other oneironauts.

Lucid Travels and the Wormhole Effect

The inspiration to pursue my dream travels in other dimensions with quantum theory happened while exploring the work of physicist Michio Kaku.[13] His explanation of quantum mechanics was eerily similar to the experiences I was having during the lucid dreaming state. In my lucid experiences, I was given superpowers in the forms of telepathy, flight, manifestation, precognition of events, and heightening of the senses. I could also travel between worlds using portals, wormholes, and membranes. I visited the underworld; flew into the eeriness of the void, where all dream imagery falls away and what is left is infinite space; and played in the imaginal realm: the place of my imagination. I met friends from parallel universes and visited relatives "from the other side."

Dr. Kaku writes about this in his work, "Blackholes, Wormholes and the Tenth Dimension." What lies on the other side of a black hole? If someone foolishly fell into a black hole, would they be crushed by its immense gravity, as most physicists believe, or would they be propelled into a parallel universe or emerge in another time era? To solve this complex question, physicists are opening up one of the most bizarre and tantalizing chapters in modern physics. They have to navigate a minefield of potentially explosive theories, such as the possibility of "wormholes," "white holes," time machines, and even the 10th dimension![14]

These are not new theories. In 1935, physicists Albert Einstein and Nathan Rosen used the theory of general relativity to propose the existence of "bridges" through space-time. These paths, called Einstein-Rosen bridges or wormholes, connect two different points in space-time, theoretically creating a shortcut that could reduce travel time and distance.[15] When Dr. Kaku elaborated on this theory of membranes, vibrations, and wormholes, it felt extremely validating. I was actually experiencing these theoretically explained phenomena in the dreamtime, and I thought: "The physicist and the oneironaut need to get together!"

In 2014, at the International Association for the Study of Dreams' annual conference in Berkeley, California, a panel titled "Gateways, Portals and Wormholes in Dreams: Bridges to Other Dimensions of Consciousness," consisting of myself, physics professor Don Middendorf and psychologists Mary Ziemer and Nigel Hamilton, explored this phenomenon of portals in dreams through different lenses and looked at how it relates to quantum mechanics, particularly wormholes.[16]

Don Middendorf writes: "Wormhole or portal or gateway dreams may often be metaphorical and personal, but they may also have an interpersonal or transpersonal component. . . . And they may be both metaphorical and have actual connections with other portions of our being or with our probable realities or other 'dimensions'."[17]

The confluence of material on this panel not only gave us a meeting point but a fascinating argument emerged: What if lucid dreams actually *create* wormholes due to a combination of observation and intention (choices)?

Middendorf also stated that:

Modern physics suggests there's no clear division of subjective and objective or 'observer' self and objects and the experience (observation) depends on our choices. Modern psychology suggests that our beliefs play a strong role in our perception and experience. Lucid dreams give us practice with both choices and beliefs and facilitate communication and harmony (alignment) with inner portions of our being or the source of consciousness.[18]

Lucid dreamers and authors, Robert Waggoner and Caroline McCready, also explore the idea of "unlimited intent" in lucid dreaming at length, as the ultimate experience, in their book *Lucid Dreaming: Plain and Simple*. "The real magic of intent occurs when you modify this process and explore open or unlimited intent . . . you do not specify the exact nature of the experience . . . [this] takes the lucid dreaming you beyond your waking knowledge."[19]

Stephen LaBerge in his book *Lucid Dreaming* reported his most satisfying lucid dreaming experiences happened when he surrendered, "suddenly he (LaBerge) found himself flying through space, past religious symbols, to a 'vast mystical realm' filled with love."[20] This would explain why children are more open to these experiences than adults, depending on the influence of perspective, culture, and belief systems.

Children's Psi Dreams and Case Studies

Lucid Dreams, OBE, and Traveling to Other Worlds

In the 1930s Carl Jung began an intensive four-year seminar on childhood dreams as recalled by adults at the Swiss Federal Institute of Technology in Zurich. Decades later, these findings were published as *Children's Dreams*[21] and have become an important document not only in the field of child development but also in the field of dream research. For Jung, children's dreams are not based on ego or the personal but "are rooted in the collective unconscious and are uprooted from it by the flood of impressions from the outside."[22]

This is why it is not unusual when many adults report they lose their imagination, including dream recall and lucid dreaming abilities, as they get older. What is also interesting to note is the pattern of these dreams in terms of content, namely extraordinary dreams.

Educational psychologist Kate Adams, at Bishop Grosseteste University in the United Kingdom, has done in-depth research on the spiritual dimensions of children's big dreams. Adams states themes like visiting heaven and angels are a common feature in children's dreams in research that spans decades. She cites C. W. Kimmins work in the 1930s. Kimmins, who studied 4,861 dreams from children aged five to eighteen, said this was particularly the case for girls aged twelve to thirteen. In her own case studies of 66 children aged nine to eleven, from both Christian and secular homes, Adams cites that a fifth of her own cases involved spiritual/religious themes. One child, Bridie, "travelled to heaven which had 'big gold gates and there was just loads and loads of little bits with beds in,' and a shop selling 'spirit candy'—sweets for spirits to buy when they go to heaven."[23]

Caroline McCready, who speaks of her own childhood adventures in lucidity, reminisces fondly of her adventures with Superman who, like in the 1978 film with Lois Lane, takes her flying. Later McCready learns that she can do the flying herself without the help of her alien friend.

> I subsequently discovered that I didn't need Superman to fly me around at all, since I could soar like a bird solo. I regularly flew over valleys, rivers and mountains. My favorite place to fly became Lake Louise in Canada, where my family used to visit … it felt amazing to be able to visit realistic dream replicas of places there, let alone fly over these magnificent landscapes.[24]

McCready also points out that, as she got older, these dreams began to dissipate. It was not until many years later that she began lucid dreaming again, and it was like "rediscovering a lost love."

Kelly Bulkeley and Patricia Bulkley's book *Children's Dreams: Understanding the Most Memorable Dreams and Nightmares of Childhood*, inspired by Carl Jung's "Children's Dreams" symposium, explores the vast dreaming terrain of childhood through case studies and psychoeducation. In one case they cite Hector, a nine year old who shares this dream:

> *I came home and my parents were sleeping in my bed. I went to my bedroom and saw myself sleeping in my bed. I left the room and the dream started all over again ... I felt weird.*[25]

The authors write that Hector was probably experiencing a lucid dream. "Many people say they had lucid dreams frequently as children but then lost the ability when they grew up, now they no longer have such dreams."[26]

Sometimes our children might dream of the deceased in another realm. This is the case of 11-year-old Claire whose friend Susie had died when the girls were both eight years old. Kate Adams reports in her book *Unseen Worlds* that Claire had a dream where she was "walking through a large gold tunnel. At the end of the tunnel she saw Susie and they engaged in conversation about their lives. Susie explained that she was happy and had made new friends whilst Claire told her about events at school."[27]

There are many research cases of OBEs in children, often connected with severe illnesses and/or Near Death Experiences (NDE); those who were pronounced clinically dead but came back to life. This was the case for Robert Moss. In his recent memoir *The Boy Who Died and Came Back*, Moss speaks candidly about how he died twice and recounts his adventures "through the Moongate." There are terms for someone like this in some cultures. In Tibet, the term is *delog*, and it refers to someone who leaves the body seemingly dead, travels in other worlds, and comes back with firsthand knowledge of the geography and current conditions in those realms. Moss does not like to label his experiences as NDEs but rather "as a boy who died and came back."[28]

Moss concludes: "... [w]hat Western psychiatry may call dissociation, ancient and indigenous cultures respect as an engagement with the Otherworld and possibly a shamanic initiation. I could step in and out of time, visit the future, and receive visitors from other times and other dimensions."[29]

Dreams of the Past, Dreams of the Future

It is not uncommon for children to dream of the past and of the future. Here is just one of the many dreams recorded that focuses on traveling to ancestral places through the river of time. The authors of *Children's Dreams* write that this was a recurring dream that began when Francine was five years old and continued for many years afterwards.

> I was a black man about twenty years old. I remember clearly what I look like, all the physical details: Tall, muscular, like an African American, definitely not a black from East Africa. I was held on a wheel, a big one in wood. They had attached my wrists and ankles and I would sink into the water of a river, rolling into the water. . . . On the other side of the river there were people singing gospel, praying for me, other black people, my friends and my family, and probably others I did not know. A special voice, so beautiful and so pure, was the one I really remember . . . I knew she was my mother, a big and powerful African woman . . . I knew I would die, everybody knew as well, they were singing for me to alleviate my pain. I would wake up very sad, suffocating as if I had water in my lungs, drowning.[30]

Francine told her mother about the dream but, because of her mother's fearful reaction, "began pretending that the dreams had stopped."[31] This is a perfect illustration of how a parent's negative reaction can deeply influence a child's willingness to share in the future; an enormous burden for a child to bear. If we can hold big dreams like this with openness instead of fear and/or dismissal, it can build trust and lead to much more insight. The authors of *Children's Dreams* observed that there are certainly larger themes here at play that "wrestle with deep questions far beyond the sphere of children's ordinary waking lives."[32] They speculate that perhaps this is also the story of the collective, the wheel of time and that Francine "remains connected to the uplifting power of her ancestral heritage, and her dreams show her the spiritual lineage of life-affirming relationships that will continue beyond her death."[33]

Studies of children's dreams and the possibility of remembering past lives have been spearheaded by Ian Stevenson, a psychiatrist and professor for the University of Virginia School of Medicine. His international recognition stemmed from his research into reincarnation through evidence suggesting that both memories and physical injuries are carried over from one lifetime to another.

Dr. Stevenson's book *Children Who Remember Previous Lives: A Question of Reincarnation*, was the result of a 40-year investigation of 3,000 cases of children around the world who recalled having past lives. From this meticulous work, Stevenson discovered a pattern of "Five Common Characteristics" of children remembering a past life.[34] Like five-year-old Francine's dream of her drowning death on the wheel, many of Stevenson's case studies reflected sudden death, whether from accidents, murder, or suicide.

He noted that 35 percent of the cases who experienced a traumatic or unnatural death had developed a phobia.[35] Francine also had a fear of water.[36]

There have been case studies of dreams of the future as well. We call these precognitive or "precog," and this means dreaming of an actual event (most likely traumatic) that occurred or will occur in waking life. In Brenda Mallon's *Dream Time with Children: Learning to Dream, Dreaming to Learn* she explores the case of Anna, a 10-year-old who dreams "mainly about the future" or what she calls "my Forward-in-Time Dreams."[37] The dream content is described as more "trivial" and personal, mainly concerning Anna's family, which Mallon states is quite common in psychic dreams.

Another case is of Delia recalling her earliest precognitive dream. It was of her mother's future hysterectomy where she was kept in the hospital and away from Delia for a long period of time because children were not allowed to visit:

> *I was 8 at the time and vividly remember a very disturbing dream in which my mother was screaming and there were several surgeons and lots of light in an operating theatre. I was watching but held away from her.*[38]

What's also interesting to note is that Delia reported that she and her mother both "have precognitive dreams regularly (and) it is discussed a lot in our home." This is also the case with Anna, who shares that it is her father who listens to her dreams and is the only one who "takes her seriously."[39] Both Mallon and Stevenson agree that culture plays a significant role in whether dreams are accepted and "taken seriously" or not. But what is certainly true of any community is that that we need to hold space for our children's dreams. This is especially important if the dream content is disturbing and involving great injury or death to a loved one.

Secrets of the Universe

Oneironauts not only travel to other worlds and through time and space, they also bring back wisdom. Lucid dream researcher Dr. Clare Johnson's daughter Yasmin reported the following dream when she was five:

> *I dreamed everybody's dreams last night—your dreams, Daddy's dreams, Oma's dreams. And I dreamed about a time when all the children were babies. And I dreamed the Earth, how it will be tomorrow.*

Clare writes:

Yasmin's dream came at around the time she started to ask me existential questions such as "Where is the universe?" "What is energy?" "Who made all the people?" (How did humanity come into existence?) "What happens when we die?" "What are dreams made of?" "Who made up all the words?" (How did language evolve?) She's been lucid dreaming since she turned three and possibly even earlier. Transcendental and spiritual lucid dream experiences can inspire people of all ages to question the nature of the universe.[40]

Bulkeley and Bulkley also cite existential dreams from children. The first dream was from an eight-year-old girl named Trudy.

I can only remember a huge dark sky filled with lots of stars. This dream recurred many times and what I remember most was the feeling it left me with every time. I felt very small and insignificant in relation to the stars.[41]

This dream was recalled from fantasy writer, John Gordon, also eight years old at the time of these dreams:

I pick up a large object far too big for me to physically lift and it is two things at once; it is vast and it is heavy and it is tiny and weightless. It is very distinctly both things yet both occupying the same space. It feels as though I hold the secret of the universe and it is the dream I believe in.[42]

What is important to note is the deep impact and influence this dream had on Gordon, whose writing profession reflects his curiosity and awe of the secrets of the universe. We can also imagine Yasmin's and Trudy's genius and life's trajectory as their big dreams are being listened to and held sacred. This is clear when we explore other famous oneironauts whose rich dream life clearly shaped their destinies and calling.

Famous Dream Travelers

Nicola Tesla and Teresa Urrea are household names, yet very few of us realize that they were true oneironauts, and that their nightly sojourns paved the way for creative thought, societal reforms, and global change.

Nikola Tesla

Inventor and genius, Nikola Tesla, was a skillful dream traveler in his youth. In his book *My Inventions: The Autobiography of Nikola Tesla*, Tesla speaks about his experiences as an oneironaut and documents them with great delight:

"Every night, (and sometimes during the day), when alone," he says, "I would start on my journeys—see new places, cities and countries; live there, meet people and make friendships and acquaintances and, however unbelievable, it is a fact that they were just as dear to me as those in actual life, and not a bit less intense in their manifestations. This I did constantly until I was about seventeen, when my thoughts turned seriously to invention."[43] What is even more astounding is Tesla's emphasis that the importance of his early childhood dream (journeys), though raw and undisciplined, shaped who he was and his work as an inventor; just as James Hillman describes the "Soul's Calling." Tesla also realized that, if he had had support and a context for his dreams earlier in life, he would not have suppressed these experiences; it would have only augmented his gifts to the world.

Tesla writes: "Those early impulses, though not immediately productive, are of the greatest moment and may shape our very destinies. Indeed, I feel now that had I understood and cultivated instead of suppressing them, I would have added substantial value to my bequest to the world. But not until I had attained manhood did I realize that I was an inventor."[44]

Teresa Urrea

In his epic book *The Hummingbird's Daughter*, Luis Urrea, author and Pulitzer Prize finalist, breathes to life the story of his Yaqui ancestor Teresa "Teresita" Urrea, also known as "Saint Teresa of Cabora." Teresa's fame and adoration blossomed during the Mexican Revolution when she was just 19 years old. What inspired Urrea to write her story was an aunt's casual remark. "You know you've got a Yaqui aunt? She can fly, goddammit! She can heal the goddamn sick and raise the dead!"[45]

Though the book is a work of fiction, Urrea conducted 20 years of meticulous research on this extraordinary revolutionary including her miraculous healing abilities, and dream traveling gifts. Here is a passage from the book that highlights Teresa's gift to leave her body and astral travel as instructed by her guardian, a medicine woman named Huila:

> When you wake up crying, Huila said, you have been there. When you wake up laughing. When the dead come to you. ... When you dream of hummingbirds. ... When your ancestors come for you and you travel with them to another town. When your dead father forgives you; when your dead mother embraces you. When you wake up and smell a foreign odor in your bedroom, a strange perfume, or smoke, or a scent of mysterious flowers, then you have been there.[46]

Tools and Tips to Help Children

Do Not Dismiss the Dream

In Kate Adams's book *Unseen Worlds* one sees the importance of her research as receiver of children's dreams. Many young people in her case studies "retreated into a world of silence until a researcher with a genuine interest came along."[47] This is the first and most important tool. Listen without judgment. When we provide a safe space for our children to talk freely, and give them our attention and care, this builds trust, connection, and confidence. Most importantly, we want our children to feel safe to come to us for help and guidance.

Seek Other Perspectives

We must not make our own interpretations of our children's dreams. Adams cites six-year-old Joe's experience when he reports "dreaming that he was on another planet playing games with some furry alien creatures. He maintains that the aliens were friendly and had promised he would visit them next week. Joe insists that he really had traveled to their land and hadn't just dreamt it."[48]

Adams points out that Joe's mother dismissed this dream as "day residue," because they had watched a film with furry aliens the day before. If the mother had instead engaged with Joe using a more psychoanalytic approach she would have gained greater insight into Joe's world.[49] Adams goes on to say if Joe was from another culture, where the belief is that the soul does indeed travel to different realms, the holding of the dream would be quite different. To honor our children's dreams we must be open to different perspectives and also allow our children to express themselves fully and freely.

Be Curious! Ask Open-Ended Questions! Invite Creativity

Rather than inserting our own opinions on what we think our children's dreams mean, we should instead be open and curious. In Joe's case we might ask him to describe the planet and the creatures that he visited. We could also ask him to express his emotions about how he felt being there playing with these friendly creatures. What activities would he like to experience when he visits the aliens again next week? By engaging with the dream we are validating the experiences while gaining new insight and connections with our children. For smaller children like Joe, we can invite them to draw the planet and the creatures or act out the dream using costumes, face painting and mask making.

Provide Dream Journals for Children

By keeping a dream journal we are in turn honoring and encouraging the dream. A blank-paged artist's sketchbook is a good choice because it evokes freedom to use the imagination. Encourage children to sketch, color, paint, collage, illustrate, or write down the dreams using poetry, prose, or myth. Robert Moss's reason to journal is "to keep a record of my experiences in the multiverse and to grow the practice of traveling to other realms and bringing back gifts."[50] By inviting in creativity, we are in fact nurturing our future superheroes, budding artists, scientists, and world leaders. Carl Jung in his collective works *Psychological Types* describes the imagination and dreams of children as not only important but as playing a crucial part in the creativity of humankind. "The debt we owe to the play of imagination is incalculable. It is therefore short-sighted to treat fantasy, on account of its risky or unacceptable nature, as a thing of little worth."[51]

Dream Sharing as Ritual

One of the most important aspects of dream practice is to bring the dream into the world. Most indigenous cultures would agree that dreams are a significant part of bringing the community together in terms of cosmology, spiritual/personal fulfillment, problem solving, and connecting with the numinous aspects of nature. For example, dream share with your family around the breakfast table before you start the day. This creates a dreaming culture and actually elicits dream recall. Protocols for dream sharing can be found on the International Association for the Study of Dreams' website.[52]

Research Ancestral Dream Practices

Both Brenda Mallon and Ian Stevenson agree that culture plays a significant role in whether dreams are accepted and "taken seriously" or not. For example, Mallon states that many African Americans hold strong beliefs in precognitive dreams as signs of guidance and warning. In *Harriet Tubman: The Moses of Her People* Sarah Bradford cited that in 1863, during the Emancipation proclamation, the great abolitionist leader Tubman was "completely calm; because, she said, she had already celebrated three years earlier when she dreamt 'My people are free! My people are free!'"[53] If you do not know your indigenous ancestry, it might be fun to research this together with your child and see what dreaming practices your ancestors used. We also have to be mindful that we do not put too much of our own beliefs in the dreams of our children. As Adams reported, many of her cases of religion and spirituality dreams came from secular households.

Reassurance for Difficult Dreams

But what is certainly true of any community or culture is the need to hold space for our children's dreams. This is especially important if the dream content is disturbing and involves great injury or death to a loved one. Mallon also points out those children who have reported precognitive dreams do not always wish to have them, as in the case of nine-year-old Rachel who stated: "I have dreams that come true and I don't like it." Brenda Mallon writes: "The best way to confront this anxiety is to assure children that though some people do have precognitive dreams, it is fairly unusual: and they can be very useful."[54] But it is also important to note that even if we find the content of the dream upsetting, it might not be a big deal for our children. Follow their lead; let them know they are safe and loved and that you will face it together.

Encouragement Through Reading

If your superhero is experiencing extraordinary dreams and, like Dr. Clare Johnson's daughter Yasmin, is starting to ask those existential questions about the nature of the universe, why not encourage her through reading? In the Further Resources section of this book, you will find a list of books for all different age groups that spark creativity and the imagination and encourage wonderment.

We as parents and caregivers, educators, and health professionals, or anyone of influence, owe it to our children to hold space for these extraordinary dreams, not only for our children's health and well-being but for that of the community. For these children are our future spiritual and political leaders, the urban mystics and scientists, the movers and the shakers: they are the future superheroes of the Dreamtime.

Notes

1. Linda Mastrangelo, "Alice's Looking Glass: Exploring Portals to Other Dimensions in Lucid Dreaming," (IASD's Psiber Dreaming Conference, 2013), 1.

2. Carl G. Jung, *Children's Dreams: Notes from the Seminar Given in 1936–1940* (Princeton, NJ: Princeton University Press, 2008).

3. Kate Adams, *Unseen Worlds: Looking through the Lens of Childhood* (London, UK, Jessica Kingsley Publishers, 2010).

4. Ibid., 160.

5. James Hillman, *The Soul's Code: In Search of Character and Calling* (New York: Random House, 1996), 3.

6. Ibid.

7. C. G. Jung, *Memories, Dreams, Reflections* (London, UK: Collins and Routledge, 1963), 356.

8. Linda Mastrangelo, "Meeting the Psychopomp: An Oneironaut's Journey into the Underworld" (IASD's Psiber Dreaming Conference, 2014), 1.

9. C. G. Jung, "ETH Lectures" (Swiss Federal Institute for Technology, July 12, 1935), 241.

10. Rudolph Steiner, *Inner Nature of Man and Life between Death and Rebirth* (New York: Anthrosophic Press, 1928).

11. Marie Jean Leon d'Hervey de Saint-Denys, *Les Rêveset les Moyens de les Diriger—Observations Pratiques* (Paris: Éditions Oniros, 1995 [1867]).

12. Robert Waggoner and Caroline McCready, *Lucid Dreaming: Plain and Simple* (San Francisco, CA: Conari Press), 1.

13. Michio Kaku, "Blackholes, Wormholes and the Tenth Dimension," accessed September 18, 2015, http://mkaku.org/home/articles/blackholes-wormholes-and-the-tenth-dimension/.

14. Ibid.

15. Michio Kaku, *Parallel Worlds: A Journey through Creation, Higher Dimensions, and the Future of the Cosmos* (Anchor, 2004), 120–121.

16. Nigel Hamilton, Linda Mastrangelo, Don Middendorf, and Mary Ziemer "Gateways, Portals and Wormholes in Dreams: Bridges to Other Dimensions of Consciousness" (Berkeley, CA: IASD Conference, 2014).

17. Don Middendorf "Wormholes and Portals as Objects and Metaphors" from "Gateways, Portals and Wormholes in Dreams" panel (Berkeley, CA: IASD Conference, 2014), 31.

18. Ibid.

19. Waggoner and McCready, *Lucid Dreams*, 116.

20. Stephen LaBerge, *Lucid Dreaming* (Los Angeles, CA: Tarcher, 1985), 86.

21. Jung, *Children's Dreams.*

22. C. G. Jung, Emma Jung, and Toni Wolff, *A Collection of Remembrances* (San Francisco, CA: Analytical Psychology Club of San Francisco, 1982) 51–70.

23. Adams, *Unseen Worlds*, 66.

24. Waggoner and McCready, *Lucid Dreaming*, xii.

25. Kelly Bulkeley and Patricia M. Bulkley, *Children's Dreams; Understanding the Most Memorable Dreams and Nightmares of Childhood* (Lanham, Maryland: Rowman & Littlefield, 2012), 66.

26. Ibid., 69.

27. Adams, *Unseen Worlds*, 69.

28. Robert Moss, *The Boy Who Died and Came Back, Adventures of a Dream Archeologist in the Multiverse* (Novato, CA: New World Library, 2013), 4.

29. Ibid.

30. Bulkeley and Bulkley, *Children's Dreams*, 76.

31. Ibid.

32. Ibid.

33. Ibid.

34. Ian Stevenson, *Children Who Remember Previous Lives: A Question of Reincarnation* (Charlottesville: The University Press of Virginia, 1987).

35. Ibid.

36. Bulkeley and Bulkley, *Children's Dreams*, 76.

37. Brenda Mallon, *Dream Time with Children; Learning to Dream, Dreaming to Learn* (London and Philadelphia: Jessica Kingsley Publishers, 2002), 164.

38. Ibid., 165.

39. Ibid.

40. Personal communication, October 2015.

41. Bulkeley and Bulkley, Children's Dreams, 100.

42. Ibid., 100–101.

43. Nikola Tesla, *My Inventions: The Autobiography of Nikola Tesla* (Eastford, CT: Martino Fine Books, 2011), 19.

44. Ibid., 6.

45. Susannah J. Felts, "My Cousin the Saint" (*Chicago Reader*, September 22, 2005). Accessed August 21, 2015, http://www.chicagoreader.com/chicago/my -cousin-the-saint/Content?oid=919991.

46. Luis Urrea, *The Hummingbird's Daughter* (New York: Back Bay Books, 2006), 126.

47. Adams, *Unseen Worlds*, 107.

48. Ibid.

49. Ibid.

50. Moss, *The Boy Who Died and Came Back*, 9.

51. Carl Jung, *Psychological Types (The Collected Works of C. G. Jung, Vol. 6) (Bollingen Series XX)* (Princeton, NJ: Princeton University Press, 1976), 82.

52. "IASD Ethical Guidelines" (International Association for the Study of Dreams) accessed July 12, 2015, http://www.asdreams.org/ethics.htm.

53. Mallon, *Dream Time with Children*, 164.

54. Ibid.

Bibliography

Adams, Kate. *Unseen Worlds: Looking through the Lens of Childhood*. London, UK: Jessica Kingsley Publishers, 2010.

Bulkeley, Kelly and Patricia M. Bulkley. *Children's Dreams; Understanding the Most Memorable Dreams and Nightmares of Childhood*. Lanham, Maryland: Rowman & Littlefield, 2012.

D'Hervey de Saint-Denys, Marie Jean Leon. *Les Rêves et les Moyens de les Diriger— Observations Pratiques*. Paris: Éditions Oniros, 1995 [1867].

Felts, Susannah J. "My Cousin the Saint" (*Chicago Reader*, September 22, 2005). Accessed August 21, 2015, http://www.chicagoreader.com/chicago/my -cousin-the-saint/Content?oid=919991.

Hamilton, Nigel, Linda Mastrangelo, Don Middendorf, and Mary Ziemer. "Gateways, Portals and Wormholes in Dreams: Bridges to Other Dimensions of Consciousness." Berkeley, CA: IASD Conference, 2014.

Hillman, James. *The Soul's Code: In Search of Character and Calling.* New York: Random House, 1996.

"IASD Ethical Guidelines" (International Association for the Study of Dreams). Accessed July12, 2015, http://www.asdreams.org/ethics.htm.

Jung, Carl G. *Children's Dreams: Notes from the Seminar Given in 1936–1940.* Princeton, NJ: Princeton University Press, 2008.

Jung, C. G. "ETH Lectures." Swiss Federal Institute for Technology, July 12, 1935, 241.

Jung, C. G. *Memories, Dreams, Reflections.* London, UK: Collins and Routledge, 1963.

Jung, Carl G. *Psychological Types. The Collected Works of C. G. Jung, Vol. 6.* Bollingen Series XX. Princeton, NJ: Princeton University Press, 1976.

Jung, C. G., Emma Jung, and Toni Wolff. *A Collection of Remembrances.* San Francisco, CA: Analytical Psychology Club of San Francisco, 1982.

Kaku, Michio. "Blackholes, Wormholes and the Tenth Dimension."Accessed September 18, 2015, http://mkaku.org/home/articles/blackholes-wormholes -and-the-tenth-dimension/.

Kaku, Michio. *Parallel Worlds: A Journey through Creation, Higher Dimensions, and the Future of the Cosmos.* New York: Anchor, 2004, 120–121.

LaBerge, Stephen. *Lucid Dreaming.* Los Angeles, CA: Tarcher, 1985, 86.

Mallon, Brenda. *Dream Time with Children; Learning to Dream, Dreaming to Learn.* London and Philadelphia: Jessica Kingley Publishers, 2002.

Mastrangelo, Linda. "Alice's Looking Glass: Exploring Portals to Other Dimensions in Lucid Dreaming." IASD's Psiber Dreaming Conference, 2013.

Mastrangelo, Linda. "Meeting the Psychopomp: An Oneironaut's Journey into the Underworld." IASD's Psiber Dreaming Conference, 2014.

Middendorf, Don. "Wormholes and Portals as Objects and Metaphors" from "Gateways, Portals and Wormholes in Dreams" panel Berkeley, CA: IASD Conference, 2014.

Moss, Robert. *The Boy Who Died and Came Back, Adventures of a Dream Archeologist in the Multiverse.* Novato, CA: New World Library, 2013.

Steiner, Rudolph. *Inner Nature of Man and Life between Death and Rebirth.* New York: Anthrosophic Press, 1928.

Stevenson, Ian. *Children Who Remember Previous Lives: A Question of Reincarnation.* Charlottesville: The University Press of Virginia, 1987.

Tesla, Nikola. *My Inventions: The Autobiography of Nikola Tesla.* Eastford, CT: Martino Fine Books, 2011.

Urrea, Luis. *The Hummingbird's Daughter.* New York: Back Bay Books, 2006.

Waggoner, Robert and Caroline McCready. *Lucid Dreaming: Plain and Simple.* San Francisco, CA: Conari Press.

CHAPTER THIRTEEN

Divine Dreams: Religious and Spiritual Themes in Children's Dreams

Kate Adams

It was dark and suddenly I saw a light, all sparkly. It was a big angel with big wings. She smiled at me and said that Nana was with her drinking a cup of tea and Nana was very happy. When I woke up, I was happy because I knew I would see Nana again one day with the angels. She always drinks tea but I don't like tea. It was a special dream.

Oliver, age 7

At times, dreams can take us by surprise. Each of us, children and adults alike, get used to particular types of dreams that we have. These include dreams about our mundane daily activities, places and people we know well, anxiety dreams about the things that concern us and, perhaps, occasional nightmares. These regular dreams are fairly easy to explain, for it is usually obvious to us how most of the imagery has arisen. But every now and then, sometimes only once or twice in a lifetime, dreams can visit us with such intensity and uniqueness that they take us unaware. Such dreams may take many forms and can have a profound, life-changing impact. Some have explicit religious content and meaning while others may have spiritual themes that are not aligned to any specific faith tradition. These dreams are often known as "divine dreams": Those in which the dreamer perceives to have a connection with a divine source and/or contain the appearance of a divine being.

The notion of some dreams having a divine connection has been with us since records began, having been reported in ancient civilizations throughout the world. Indeed, the belief that some dreams can be a means of communication with God can be found in holy texts such as the Hebrew Bible, the New Testament, and the Quran.[1] There are also contemporary commentaries on divine dreams of adults[2] but despite the fact that children also report occasional divine dreams, these are rarely researched. This is particularly interesting because it is well established that the most memorable dreams often occur in childhood[3] and can remain with us for a lifetime, often leading to reflection on life's philosophical issues and sometimes to changes in behavior and lifestyle. You would, however, be forgiven for not being aware of children's divine dreams because in many economically developed societies they are certainly not the topic of general conversation. Yet, although not widely researched, those studies that have focused solely on children's divine dreams, detailed throughout this chapter, tend to show that around a fifth of all those questioned reported one. Hence, they may not be as rare as one might first imagine.

This chapter brings to light this fascinating aspect of children's extraordinary dreaming. It is a topic close to my heart. Many people assume that my interest in it must arise from my own experience of a divine dream during childhood but actually that is not the case; I have not encountered such a dream. Instead, when I was a teacher, I was inspired by a young boy in my class who told me in some detail how God talked to him in his dreams. His story led me to undertake a small research project with children to explore the phenomenon further, which then led to me undertaking a PhD on the subject and writing a book, *Unseen Worlds: Looking through the Lens of Childhood*,[4] that explores children's dreams and nightmares alongside other elements of their worlds that adults often miss, such as imaginary friends and seeing angels. In doing so I have met many wonderful children and been honored to have them share these very special, often private, experiences with me.

This chapter draws on some of those children's narratives, alongside those who have talked to other researchers, to offer examples of a variety of children's dreams, accompanied by their own narratives about their perceived origin and meaning. In doing so, voice is given to the children because it is essential that we understand these dreams from their experiential viewpoints, as well as from an adult-centric stance. We explore the responses which adults often give to them and, crucially, what we can learn from children themselves. Suggestions for parents and caregivers are also included to help navigate this intriguing aspect of dreaming that may sit uneasily for many people. Importantly, this chapter makes no claims as to whether or not a dream can genuinely have a divine source or if a divine being can manifest in a dream; these decisions are for each individual reader to make. Instead the chapter hears and respects the voices of children and their opinions—the voices and opinions of children from religious homes as well as those from secular homes.

Types of Divine Dreams

A range of themes emerge from these extraordinary dreams, which align with various religious traditions and also with psychological studies of dream content. Perhaps the broadest categories are dreams *about* God (and occasionally another divine figure) and dreams *from* God, in which there is no actual appearance of God. The former are relatively common among children of Christian and secular backgrounds. In these cases, it is often reported that God appeared in anthropomorphic form in ways which aligned to the children's waking perceptions of what God is like—a finding from my own research conducted in England and Scotland and also by Ferdinand Potgieter, Johannes van der Walt, and Charl Wolhuter,[5] who conducted a similar study in South Africa.

In England, 11-year-old Jenny, from a secular home, dreamed of heaven, where she saw her deceased rabbit with God standing on steps made of clouds. Dressed in a long robe, and with a moustache, God took the form of a man who was crying as he welcomed Jenny in her visit to heaven to see her pet rabbit. In the dream, Jenny felt frightened but told me that God gave her comfort.

Kirsty, a nine-year-old Christian girl, described her dream figure as being bald with thick eyebrows and wearing "a skirt." In waking life she did not have a definitive view of God's demeanor but expressed surprise at the hairless figure, stating: "I don't think if I met God that He would be bald!" However, it would be a mistake to assume that all of the children's dream images of God were in such a recognizable form as Jenny and Kirsty's. For example, Ruth, also from a Christian background, saw a shadow moving clockwise around her bedroom. She thought that there was a face in it, but her recall of it was poor and she could not offer a description. However, Ruth believed that this shadow was God. She explained:

> I think he might have come as a shadow because he might have not wanted people to see his real self or what He will look like. He does want people to spread the word about Him, or His work, but I don't think He wants people

to go around going "I saw God, I saw God" ... Some people do get bullied because of their religion but I don't think God wanted that to start, so I think He might have just come as a shadow ... to protect them.

We will return to the theme of bullying later. Before, then, let us take a look at dreams that children perceive to have been sent by God. These are often less immediately obvious as "divine dreams" to the observer, and thus demonstrate the importance of listening to the child's explanation. One example is offered by Rasha, a Muslim girl, who dreamed that she and a cousin were going on Hajj. She traveled by car and watched her cousin traveling by boat. In the distance, the girls saw Mecca and the Kaaba before the boat turned around. Although the dream did not contain any images of the girls performing Hajj, Rasha had an intuitive feeling that Allah had sent this dream to her as a message instructing her to go on Hajj in the future.

Themes of Divine Dreams

Messages

Whether or not children's dreams are about or from God, common themes recur in both content and in the children's interpretation of them. Perhaps the unifying descriptor in a divine dream, which spans the majority of them, is that the children understood them to contain a message that had a divine source. This notion is inherent in scriptures from different religions, including ancient religions, Judaism, Christianity, and Islam, and cuts across all of the dreams included in this chapter, irrespective of which category they are placed in. The messages that the children report, across various studies, are all individual to them and apply to their personal life circumstances at the time of the dream.

In my own research, Martin, a 10-year-old Christian boy, recalled a dream that he had had two years previously, in which a man was praying on a hill and subsequently vanished. Martin then heard a voice, which he believed to be God's, saying, "Never let go of anyone in your family." Martin linked the dream to a family argument during which he had accused his parents of entering his bedroom against his wishes. Following the altercation, he had written a note to his parents threatening that if they did not make an admission of guilt, he would leave home. Martin believed that God's message in the dream "was kind of a reminder like your mum made you, so ... you'd be very unwise to go away." Martin explained that he decided to stay at home and value his parents more as a result of the dream.

Reassurance

Children worry about a wide range of things, from exams and falling out with friends to illness and death, and dreams can be a way of providing reassurance. Sometimes these take the form of divine dreams, as Potgieter, van der Walt, and Wolhuter[6] also found. In their South African study, reassurance was the most common dream theme reported by the 12- and 13-year-olds. These included assurance of: the existence of God (and the heavenly angels); predestination (being "chosen" by God as one of His children); a heavenly afterlife; a Godly presence (either Jesus himself, Jesus and the angels, or just the angels alone) during bad times; and that deceased loved ones were alive and well.

Undertaking research in California, Cynthia Sauln[7] reported a recurring dream narrated by a 10-year-old African American boy called Protector. It contained a combination of fearful and reassuring content. He told Sauln:

> So I'm surrounded by buildings and they just collapse and the streets start to break. I knew the end of the world isn't going to happen anytime soon, but it's like I feel like it is and I feel scared. I know it's not going to happen. I just feel scared if it does. But then I see God riding on a horse. He is riding on a horse that is on a cloud, and he picks us up and he takes us to heaven. ... Basically He didn't say anything. He doesn't talk. He just, He took up our sins and then He took us but not our sins. He took our bodies to get up to heaven. When we're there, we won't have any suffering or anything—nothing to worry about as we know He's on our side.

Protector took this dream to be a message from God that God would care for him. He was comforted by the belief that the dream showed him that God was in control and overall he need not be scared.

However, not all of these dreams have explicit religious content. One such example is the dream of Sarah, a Christian girl, who was anxious about a cross-country run at school. The night before the race, she dreamed that she ran the course without difficulty, completed it, and was not last over the finishing line. Sarah understood the dream to be an indication from God that she had the ability to run the race successfully. She explained how it led her to be less nervous about the event on the day and was ultimately relieved to have finished the course without being last.[8]

In her book *Dream Time with Children*, Brenda Mallon[9] cites a 13-year-old boy who described how he had been ill when he was 5 years old. During his illness, he dreamed that an angel entered his room to talk to his mother. His mother explained to the angel that her son was ill and the angel blessed him. In the dream, his illness was instantly cured. Dreams such as this can offer children feelings of reassurance on awakening—not only in the resolution of a problem but also comfort that there is a greater power taking care of them.

Clinical psychologist Patricia Garfield,[10] in her book *The Universal Dream Key*, describes how dreams of loss and death are considered "universal dreams," appearing across all cultures. Often, such dreams also fall into the category of divine dreams and can give reassurance, as Samantha, aged 10, described. She came from a family who were occasional churchgoers. The dream came at a time when her father had taken her pet hamster, named Hammy, to the vet. In the dream, an angel told her that:

> *Hammy would be happier and he would be looked after well and he wouldn't feel any pain or anything.*

Samantha understood this to mean that Hammy would soon die, but that he would have a better life after his physical death. However, this information contradicted her father's words of compassion that followed his visit to the vet: "I said to Dad, 'I think [Hammy's] going to die,' and Dad said 'don't worry.' But I don't think I am that stupid actually."

The dream proved to be accurate, overriding her father's opinion, and Hammy soon died, yet Samantha found the dream reassuring. Although naturally saddened by losing her pet, Samantha was pleased that the angel had informed her of his death "in a nice way." This had given her "an extra boost." She explained: "It makes me feel a lot happier 'cos sometimes I feel upset about [Hammy's death] but when I think about the dream I feel a lot happier." Further, it had helped her to console her younger siblings by assuring them that Hammy would be living a blissful life after his bodily death.[11]

Dreaming the Future

A further recurring theme, found in my research and to a lesser extent in Potgieter, van der Walt, and Wolhuter's[12] study was dreaming of the future. Interestingly, such "precognitive" dreams are a feature of scripture (e.g., the dreams of Joseph/Yusuf in the Hebrew Bible and Quran predicting years of feast and famine and his rise to power in Egypt) and are also a recognized phenomenon in psychological literature. The key element for children's divine dreams is that the perceived vision of the future is not necessarily of a religious or spiritual happening. Often, the prediction may be related to a secular matter but the children believe that the source of the dream was God. Ahmed, a Muslim boy from Scotland, told me of his dream:

I was on my bike going down the hill [on the road where I live] and the bike was going really fast. Then suddenly straight ahead of me was a tree. I was going to crash into it but then I swerved and just missed it! And the next day it really happened.

To the listener, this may seem like an ordinary dream, located in Ahmed's daily context and activities. But through talking to Ahmed I learned that there was much more to the dream than was initially apparent. He went on to explain how a few days later he had been riding his bike down the hill when he suddenly realized he was about to hit the tree. Having had the dream, he knew exactly what to do: slam on his brakes. He did so, and stopped ahead of the tree, thereby avoiding an injury. For Ahmed, the dream had predicted this event but at first I was still unable to ascertain how this might be a divine dream. But Ahmed explained all:

"This dream came from Allah." he said.
"How do you know it was Allah?" I asked.
"Only Allah knows the future!" he replied.

Through our conversation, it also became apparent that the dream was a sign for Ahmed that Allah was protecting and guiding him and hence the dream offered him reassurance and security.[13]

Eight-year-old Michael reported a dream that predicted the future but at the same time offered him reassurance. He dreamed that he was on holiday with his father at a theme park, where he was about to go on a frightening ride called "Vertical Limit." The ride involved plunging down a steep chute into a pool of water. In the dream, Michael was terrified but he heard a voice saying, "stop panicking, have more faith and more confidence." He told me how the dream manifested when his father took him on a surprise holiday, during which he found himself facing the challenge of the ride. Not only did he overcome his fear and go down the chute, but also gained increased self-confidence as a result of doing so. He explained how the dream was unusual for him because it was not a nightmare.

Darker Dreams

It would be to do a disservice to children, and adults, to suggest that all divine dreams are enlightening, reassuring, mystical, magical, or numinous experiences that offer profound insights into meaning and purpose and a sense of a caring and protective higher power. A smaller number are somewhat more unsettling, or even frightening. This is not unsurprising given that psychologists have clearly shown that nightmares are a normal part of childhood[14] though this fact may come as little comfort to the child or to their worried parents and other caregivers. But, as Alan Siegel and Kelly Bulkeley[15] observe, children can find many aspects of religion quite frightening, such as rituals, dramatic stories, and myths. They describe the nightmare of Lucy, a seven-year-old girl who lived in a Hindu community and who was frightened by the adults' white robes. She had a nightmare in which one of the Hindu worshippers appeared in her room. In the dream she ran and ran in fear and finally woke up screaming. Her parents were able to resolve her fears by taking her to meet a Hindu elder who explained about the religion, which subsequently relieved her anxieties. This is a helpful example of how adults can support children when their dreams are unsettling—a theme that is explored further toward the end of the chapter.

It is not uncommon to dream of death, irrespective of age. Denise, a Christian girl, dreamed that she was on a mountain and slipped. She told me how she had fallen off the mountain:

> and then the next thing I knew I was in what I thought was heaven and there was these big gold and silvery sparkly gates in front of me and they opened and there was God and Jesus standing there.

Denise was initially shaken by the dream—the only time she had dreamed of her own death—but was also comforted by the fact that she went to heaven.

Adults' Responses

When a child shares a divine dream with an adult, they report a range of responses. Naturally, these will depend upon the context, not least on whether the adult being told is a parent, grandparent, child-minder, religious leader, teacher, or other professional. The response will also be shaped by the cultural context and the disposition of the adult. Are they religious? Do they have time to listen and talk through the dream? Are they open to the idea of divine dreams or might they see such experiences as indicative of a vivid imagination or even a mental illness?

However, there is a common thread running through children's views on how their divine dream had been received by adults; namely that a significant proportion of those who chose to share their dream received a negative reaction. Most commonly, children are told "it's just your imagination," which they take to be a complete dismissal of their experience. At times, perhaps adults say this because they are uncomfortable with the account of the dream. Perhaps they do not know how to respond. Perhaps they are nervous that the child is making up stories to gain attention, or that there may be some more worrying element at play such as mental illness particularly if a child is persistent in talking about such dreams. In other cases, children have explained that adults have laughed at them, or have taken no interest at all. Perhaps these scenarios arise because adults are uneasy with the concept, or are simply too busy to listen rather than not being interested. Whatever the case, children have been left feeling dismissed. That is a lonely place for a child to be. Other children, who have not disclosed their dream to anyone other than a researcher, have done so for fear of a negative response. That too is a lonely place for a child to be.

But adults who do not react with interest are not the only group of people who can proffer negative responses. Other children can too. Earlier, Ruth made a reference to people being "bullied for their religion" but some children also fear being bullied for talking about dreams. In one school I visited in Scotland, a teacher advised me that one of her students had declined to take part in my research even though he had a dream about God, because he "knew that if he came to see me, the other children in the class would know that he had a dream, and they would pick on him." Similarly, in South Africa, children said that they could not inform their peers about their dream.[16] The authors cite a pertinent comment from one of the girls: "I am captain of the first Netball team. Can you imagine what the parents of my friends would say if they knew? How can someone who claims to have had a dream in which angels had appeared to her be allowed to lead the School's Netball team?"

Such responses are not unsurprising. David Hay,[17] writing on religion and spirituality in the West, interviewed adults and found that many, particularly men, are reluctant to share their spiritual experiences because the West has a "suspicion of the spiritual." Such a culture is inevitably learned by children at a relatively young age. It lies in stark contrast with findings from some anthropological studies that show how some cultures highly value dreams. For example, Kelly Bulkeley[18] describes the beliefs of the Mekeo people in New Guinea who regard dreams as occurring when the dream-self leaves the body during sleep to travel to the places seen in the dream. There, dreams are highly valued as a means of gaining spiritual power. While the community sees many dreams as being relatively trivial, others are very powerful and interpretation is required to fully understand their meaning. Clearly, in a culture such as that of the Mekeo, a child's dream would likely be accorded more respect than in a culture which gives them less credence.

It is also essential to emphasize that many children may not want to share their divine dream, and their right not to is always to be respected. Adults need to avoid the temptation to draw experiences out of children; to do so can not only put undue pressure on them but also potentially lead them to fabricate dreams simply to satisfy the adults in question. Both scenarios are of course unethical.

How Can Adults Respond to Children's Divine Dreams?

Listening without Judgment

Given that a divine dream may hold great significance for the child, possibly being one which will remain with them for a lifetime, particular sensitivities are needed for engaging with their experiences. As a researcher I play a specific role, which has elements that are applicable for all adults engaging with children and their dreams in any walk of life. One is to listen . . . and to listen without judgment. Children are very sensitive to being judged and can intuit insincerity quickly. Being a researcher is a privileged role in many ways, because the children know in advance that they will be taken seriously; the researcher is a person who is meeting them to genuinely learn about their views, offer assurances of confidentiality and the pair may not meet again. This distance between the adult and child can enable the child to be more open, knowing that they will be taken seriously.

For parents and other adults close to the child, the same principle of listening without judgment applies. But this is not always as easy as it may sound under the circumstances of close relationships, particularly if a family has no specific religious orientation. In such cases it may come as a shock to hear one's son or daughter talking about a divine dream, but this is not actually unsurprising, since religious language—God, heaven, angels—is commonplace in society. Children see and hear it in television programs such as *The Simpsons* and comments by adults who, for example, might seek to reassure children after bereavement with words such as "Grandma has gone to heaven," even if that may not be the view of the adult.

In many schools, particularly in Europe, Religious Education is a part of the curriculum, so religious language is not only known by children but also used by them. A child's use of religious language may be a means of exploring their sense of meaning and purpose in the world—something which all children do—and in this case, doing so through the medium of their dreams. Depending on the circumstances, some children may be "thinking out loud" and not actually be seeking a discussion. In other cases, they may feel a need to talk through the experience of the dream and their reflections on it, especially if it occurred as a nightmare.

Dream Sharing

The concept of listening to a child's thoughts about a dream is closely linked to the practice of dream sharing, which Alan Siegel and Kelly Bulkeley[19] describe in their very readable book *Dreamcatching: Every Parent's Guide to Exploring and Understanding Children's Dreams and Nightmares.*

They offer guidelines on how to share dreams with children in a family context, which involves the following stages:

- **Welcoming the dream**
  Create an atmosphere in which dreams are valued and children are encouraged to share them in the home, but resist the temptation to interpret them.
- **Telling and retelling the dream**
  Encourage children to tell and retell the dream in the first person ("I") and in the present tense to make the dream more "real."
- **Empathizing with feelings in the dream**
  In order to understand the child's perspective, especially if they are young and are having difficulty in articulating it, introduce the phrase "if it were my dream" to help uncover the child's perspective and in turn to be able to empathize with them more effectively.
- **Breaking the spell of bad dreams**
  When a child is distressed, offer physical and verbal reassurances and let them know that you have also had bad dreams. Acknowledge how frightening they can be. Ask your child questions about the dream to help them learn more about their inner world.

Although not specifically linked to divine dreams, their advice holds true for this type of extraordinary dream, as do the following approaches, all of which may need to be supplemented by specific discussion about the religious or spiritual dimensions of the dream.

Writing and Artwork

Authors who write about working with children's dreams and nightmares[20] all refer to the valuable use of representing the dreams and, where appropriate, their alternative endings. This can be achieved through writing and various forms of artwork such as drawings, paintings, or collage. These processes can help clarify the dream for both child and adult, facilitate seeing it from different perspectives, and foster a listening environment.

Nightmares

Of course, when divine dreams become dark and manifest as nightmares, there is a particular urgency for parents and children to find resolution. Writing on nightmares more generally, Ann Sayre Wiseman[21] focuses on practical strategies to help children deal with their nightmares. She asks them to draw the dream, the act of which places a child in control. She ensures that the child feels safe enough to reenter the nightmare and if they are too frightened to recall it, she encourages them to create ways of empowering themselves. Strategies include drawing a shield, capturing a monster in a cage or creating an army of friends to help them become invisible. The next stage is to encourage the child to talk to the monster/frightening figure and ask why it has come, which gives a child authority over it. Wiseman proposes that children negotiate with the character rather than simply trying to destroy it and argues that children should be encouraged to find creative resolutions, thereby empowering them.[22]

Siegel and Bulkeley[23] describe a method entitled The Four Rs that involves:

- Reassurance
- Rescripting
- Rehearsal
- Resolution

Reassurance involves recognition of the emotional and physical elements, and encourages the child to feel safe to discuss their nightmare. Rescripting particularly focuses on creating a new ending for the dream, perhaps through writing or artwork, and rehearsal involves repeating the dream and its possible solutions until the child feels that they have mastered the rescripting. Finally, the resolution can come once the origin of the dream has been acknowledged and the solution mastered.

When such aforementioned techniques are applied to divine dreams, there may be additional complexities, particularly for religious families who struggle to understand why their child is frightened by aspects of their faith. Again, this process will rely on careful listening and trying to empathize with how they are feeling; on seeing the world through the child's eyes.

Learning from Children

There is much to be learned from listening to children's divine dreams. The first relates to how open children are to worlds that we may refer to as "unseen."[24] These unseen worlds extend way beyond dreams, to other elements that adults may have encountered in their own childhoods but may have lost sight of since. These include having imaginary friends, seeing the guardian angel at the foot of the bed or seeing spirits of people who have passed away. Many children certainly appear to have an innate heightened sense of awareness of realms, which adults cannot access or categorize as "imagination" that seems to decrease rapidly with age.

Second, the examples of the dreams given here show how many children have a natural ability to find meaning in their dreams. Never in my own research have I asked children for an interpretation of their dream, for that would be a leading question. Instead I only asked them what they thought made that dream a divine one, or to explain why they thought they had had the dream. Yet children spontaneously offered quite detailed responses, which demonstrated that not only had they already intuitively found meaning in the dream, but some of those meanings were sophisticated. Herein lies a warning not to overlook what may first appear to be a "bland" dream. While the content may well seem relatively easy to explain, such as it being related to a concern or anxiety in the child's everyday life, there may well be far more depth to the dream in the child's interpretation.

Third, the only way to be certain about the perceived meaning of the dream through a child's eyes is to engage with them in exploring it—assuming of course that they wish to. The lesson to be learned from some of the children featured in this chapter is to never dismiss a dream that seems ordinary or banal, for it may nevertheless have been a significant religious or spiritual experience for the child.

Divine dreams may be treated with suspicion by many. They may be dismissed as works of imagination. Conversely they may be treated as authentic communications with a higher power. Regardless of which viewpoint you take, they have a long history throughout time across the world. But most importantly, for some children, dreams occur which they believe have a divine connection. For many who experience them, they can have a profound impact on their thinking, offer reassurance in times of worry or help them make sense of events such as death and loss.

Not all children who have divine dreams are from religious homes, but particularly for those who are, they can also offer feelings of an enhanced connection with God. Arguably, it may be a topic that some adults find less easy to discuss than children do. But given the right environment—of respect, acceptance, and nonjudgmental listening—being open to children's divine dreams can be very rewarding, and of great benefit to children who may otherwise find themselves without anyone to talk to.

Notes

1. Kelly Bulkeley, *Dreaming in the World's Religions: A Comparative History* (New York and London: New York University Press, 2008).

2. Richard Curley, "Private Dreams and Public Knowledge in a Camerounian Independent Church," in *Dreaming, Religion and Society in Africa*, edited by Marian Charles Jedrej and Rosalind Shaw (Leiden: E. J. Brill, 1992), 135–152; Simon Charsley, "Dreams in African Churches," in *Dreaming, Religion and Society in Africa*, edited by Marian Charles Jedrej and Rosalind Shaw (Leiden: E. J. Brill, 1992), 133–176.

3. Kelly Bulkeley, Bitsy Broughton, Anita Sanchez, and Joanne Stiller, "Earliest Remembered Dreams," *Dreaming* 15, no. 3 (2005): 205–222.

4. Kate Adams, *Unseen Worlds: Looking through the Lens of Childhood* (London: Jessica Kingsley, 2010).

5. Ferdinand J. Potgieter, Johannes L. van der Walt, and Charl C. Wolhuter, "The Divine Dreams of a Sample of South African Children: The Gateway to Their Spirituality," *International Journal of Children's Spirituality* 14, no. 1 (2009): 31–46.

6. Potgieter et al., "Divine Dreams," 31–46.

7. Cynthia, S. Sauln, "In My Dreams I Am the Hero I Wish to Be: A Mixed-Methods Study of Children's Dreams, Meaning Making, and Spiritual Awareness," 2013. Unpublished PhD thesis. Sofia University, accessed May 5, 2015, http://gradworks.umi.com/35/96/3596835.html.

8. Kate Adams, "Children's Dreams: An Exploration of Jung's Concept of Big Dreams," *International Journal of Children's Spirituality* 8, no. 2 (2003): 105–114.

9. Brenda Mallon, *Dream Time with Children: Learning to Dream, Dreaming to Learn* (London: Jessica Kingsley Publishers, 2002).

10. Patricia Garfield, *The Universal Dream Key: The 12 Most Common Dream Themes around the World* (New York: HarperCollins, 2001).

11. Kate Adams, Brendan Hyde, and Richard Woolley, *The Spiritual Dimension of Childhood* (London: Jessica Kingsley, 2008); Adams, *Unseen Worlds*.

12. Potgieter et al., "Divine Dreams," 31–46.

13. Adams, *Unseen Worlds*.

14. Alan Siegel and Kelly Bulkeley, *Dreamcatching: Every Parent's Guide to Exploring and Understanding Children's Dreams and Nightmares* (New York: Three Rivers Press, 1998); Mallon, *Dream Time*.

15. Siegel and Bulkeley, *Dreamcatching*.

16. Potgieter et al., "Divine Dreams," 31–46.

17. David Hay, "Suspicion of the Spiritual: Teaching Religion in a World of Secular Experience," *British Journal of Religious Education* 7, no. 3 (1985): 40–147.

18. Bulkeley, *Dreaming in the World's Religions*.

19. Siegel and Bulkeley, *Dreamcatching*.

20. Ann Sayre Wiseman, *Nightmare Help: A Guide for Parents and Teachers* (Berkeley: Ten Speed Press, 1989); Siegel and Bulkeley, *Dreamcatching*; Mallon, *Dream Time*.

21. Wiseman, *Nightmare Help*.

22. Adams, *Unseen Worlds*.

23. Siegel and Bulkeley, *Dreamcatching*.

24. Adams, *Unseen Worlds*.

Bibliography

Adams, Kate. "Children's Dreams: An Exploration of Jung's Concept of Big Dreams." *International Journal of Children's Spirituality* 8, no. 2 (2003): 105–114.

Adams, Kate. *Unseen Worlds: Looking through the Lens of Childhood.* London: Jessica Kingsley, 2010.

Adams, Kate, Brendan Hyde, and Richard Woolley. *The Spiritual Dimension of Childhood.* London: Jessica Kingsley, 2008.

Bulkeley, Kelly, Bitsy Broughton, Anita Sanchez, and Joanne Stiller. "Earliest Remembered Dreams." *Dreaming* 15, no. 3 (2005): 205–222.

Bulkeley, Kelly. *Dreaming in the World's Religions: A Comparative History.* New York and London: New York University Press, 2008.

Charsley, Simon. "Dreams in African Churches." In *Dreaming, Religion and Society in Africa.* Edited by Marian Charles Jedrej, and Rosalind Shaw, 133–176. Leiden: E. J. Brill, 1992.

Curley, Richard. "Private Dreams and Public Knowledge in a Camerounian Independent Church." In *Dreaming, Religion and Society in Africa.* Edited by Marian Charles Jedrej, and Rosalind Shaw, 135–152. Leiden: E. J. Brill, 1992.

Garfield, Patricia. *The Universal Dream Key: The 12 Most Common Dream Themes around the World.* New York: HarperCollins, 2001.

Hay, David. "Suspicion of the Spiritual: Teaching Religion in a World of Secular Experience." *British Journal of Religious Education* 7, no. 3 (1985): 40–147.

Mallon, Brenda. *Dream Time with Children: Learning to Dream, Dreaming to Learn.* London: Jessica Kingsley Publishers, 2002.

Potgieter, Ferdinand, J., Johannes L. van der Walt, and Charl C. Wolhuter. "The Divine Dreams of a Sample of South African Children: The Gateway to Their Spirituality." *International Journal of Children's Spirituality* 14, no. 1 (2009): 31–46.

Sauln, Cynthia, S. "In My Dreams I Am the Hero I Wish to Be: A Mixed-Methods Study of Children's Dreams, Meaning Making, and Spiritual Awareness." 2013. Unpublished PhD thesis. Sofia University. Accessed May 5, 2015. http://gradworks.umi.com/35/96/3596835.html.

Siegel, Alan, and Kelly Bulkeley. *Dreamcatching: Every Parent's Guide to Exploring and Understanding Children's Dreams and Nightmares.* New York: Three Rivers Press, 1998.

Wiseman, Ann Sayre. *Nightmare Help: A Guide for Parents and Teachers.* Berkeley: Ten Speed Press, 1989.

CHAPTER FOURTEEN

Dream Magicians: Empower Children through Lucid Dreaming

Clare R. Johnson

I saw the witches in my dream again but I knew it was a dream so I wasn't scared because I knew they were only lonely and wanted to be my friend, or they wanted something to eat or something to play with. So I used the Abracadabra spell to magic a witch doll for them to play with. Then the doll came alive! It was a real witch baby and the witches loved it! Then I turned them all into princesses and later on back into witches again. We all had a lovely time playing.

Yasmin Johnson, age 4

In a lucid dream, we *know* that we are dreaming *while* we are dreaming. Lucid dreaming goes beyond the imagination: It offers us new experiences that seem just as real as waking life. In lucid dreams, we can fly like Superwoman, turn into a panther, paint a door in the air and walk through it into a new dream, breathe underwater, jump over tall buildings, and float among infinite stars. We can extend and deepen our life experience while dreaming—our dreaming years do not have to be dead ones! We spend a third of our lives asleep, and an estimated six years of that time dreaming. Why not help children to turn their dreaming years into life-enhancing ones?

In lucid dreams we can be outrageously creative, playing with the impact our thoughts and intentions have on the dream environment and events.[1] We can confront nightmare images and converse with our deepest fears, waking up with a sense of release and fulfillment. We can even experience spiritual transformation. On a practical level, lucid dreamers can practice motor skills such as swimming strokes or judo kicks,[2] and wake up to find they have mastered them, as demonstrated by one talented lucid dreamer I interviewed, 10-year-old Claire Shticks:

> In gymnastics you have to learn a complicated trick called a "kip." It was taking me months to learn it when Mom suggested I practice my kip in my lucid dreams. In this particular lucid dream, gymnastics equipment is laying around in our living room. I get a dreamy feeling so I check my hands to get confirmation. I have six fingers in one hand. I get happy and I remember to try to get my kip, so I walk over to the bars and execute a perfect kip! I keep repeating the move until I wake up.
>
> The next day I was able to get my kip on the bars![3]

Why *Lucid* Dreams?

When we know that we are dreaming, we can engage consciously with the dream world, recognizing it as a malleable cocreation that is responsive to our thoughts, emotions, and intentions. We also know that this is a world from which we will wake up safely. Simply becoming lucid in a nightmare can cause all fear to vanish and in response to the dreamer's new mindset, the dreamscape may spontaneously transform into something beautiful or healing. Lucid dreaming can empower children of all ages to have a happier, more fulfilling dream life.

In a lucid dream, children can do dreamwork while in the dream. This puts them in an extremely powerful position for transformation, particularly in the area of recurring nightmares, which have been shown to respond well to lucid dreaming therapy.[4] Dreams, whether they are lucid or not, can be deeply wise, and I consider dreamplay techniques such as drawing the dream or acting it out to be forms of waking lucidity because here, too, there is a wonderful mix of conscious and unconscious. It is this mixture that makes dreamplay so effective because we are not relying simply on our logical, rational conscious mind but are fusing it with deep dream imagery straight from the unconscious. It is the same in lucid dreaming: as Charles Tart said, "The lucid dreamer wakes up in terms of mental functioning within the dreamworld."[5]

How accessible is lucid dreaming to children between the ages of two and eighteen? The answer appears to be: "Very." A 1998 study by Lapina, Lysenko, and Burikov found 80–90 percent rates of lucid dream frequency in 15- to 18-year-olds.[6] One 2006 study by Qinmei, Qinggong, and Jie shows that most four- to six-year-olds believe that there may be a way of controlling the action in their dreams, while knowing that this is a dream.[7] In very young children, the difficulty with asking them specifically about their lucid dreams lies in ensuring that they fully understand the difference between lucid and nonlucid dreams. When my daughter Yasmin was two and a quarter she began to make positive changes in her nightmares according- ing to my suggestions, but her lack of vocabulary meant it was impossible for me to ascertain whether these were fully lucid dreams or not. If you ask a child that young: "When the dragon was chasing you, did you know that it was a dream dragon?" she will nod and say "yes," but she may simply mean that she knows *now that she is awake* that the dragon appeared in a dream. By the age of three, however, Yasmin was reporting what sounded like definite lucid dreams: "This is a dream! I can do magic!"

A great many children seem to have spontaneous lucid dreams without ever having heard of "waking up inside a dream," and once they become familiar with the concept, youngsters have the ability to pick up lucid dreaming very quickly. The aforementioned study by Lapina et al. found that teaching a sample of thirteen 10- to 12-year-olds lucid dream induction techniques such as reality checks,[8] redreaming,[9] and MILD[10] (Mnemonic Induction of Lucid Dreams) over a six week period resulted in 92 percent of the children having at least one lucid dream. Such studies indicate that lucid dreaming is a learnable skill for the majority of children.

Lucid dreaming puts children in a strong position to work on their dreams and nightmares *while they are dreaming.* If children wish to guide the lucid dream, there are many possibilities for doing so in ways which encourage self-belief, creative thinking, and problem-solving skills. These skills can carry over into the child's daily life, empowering him or her both in the dream world and the waking world. Once lucid, the dreamer can become a dream magician if he or she wants to, because lucid dreaming is a highly thought-responsive environment:[11] simply thinking about something can cause it to manifest. This means being a dream magi- cian can be as simple as thinking a clear, guiding thought in a lucid dream, or it can involve more complex actions such as reciting mantras and spells, creating new dream scenes, or using magical props such as an invisibility cloak or a wishing ring.

Young children often feel powerless in their dreams, just as they do in waking life, since adults have complete control over them.[12] If children are informed about the possibilities open to them when they have a lucid dream, they can begin to take steps toward personal empowerment. This empowerment carries over into waking life situations and can help children to gain confidence and learn to speak out. This chapter discusses how to empower children in practical, lasting ways through (a) lucid dreaming and the four levels of lucid dream magic; (b) transforming bad dreams with my L.O.V.E. Nightmare Empowerment Technique; (c) dream-play as waking lucidity.

My doctoral research[13] investigated the creative possibilities open to "dream magicians":[14] those who consciously guide events and experiment with magical abilities while lucid in a dream.[15] I have developed a model for lucid dream magic according to the four levels of engagement I identified within lucid dreaming. The following tips for budding dream magicians can be adapted to any age group.

How to Be a Dream Magician

Watch Your Dream Film

This first level of lucid dream magic takes place during what I have termed Passive Observation Lucid Dreams,[16] where the dreamer watches the dream unfold without joining in. Not all lucid dreams have to involve dream control! It can be fascinating simply to watch the dream action, knowing that you will wake up safely from this experience. Just *knowing that this is a dream* can transform fear and other negative emotions instantaneously, and often the thought-responsive dream environment reacts accordingly: monsters shrink, dragons turn into sweet new friends. Lucidity can transform both the dreamer and the dream, as Ken Kelzer, author of *Lucid Dreaming: The Sun and the Shadow*, reports: "the moment that I became lucid I experienced total inner transformation. All my fear vanished in an instant, and inside of myself I felt full of courage."[17]

On this level of engagement, self-reflective knowledge is the only "magic" deployed. The dreamer recognizes: "I am dreaming!" Implicit is the understanding that he will wake up safely from this experience. With this knowledge, any fear or unease tends to vanish as curiosity and excitement take over. The dream can be watched like a film of the imagination at play. The dreamer's thoughts and emotions will have an effect on the "dream film" even if he is not physically involved in the action, so very often the dream imagery will transform according to the child's emotions and expectations. Of course, if the child becomes lucid during a nightmare that feels too frightening to stay in, he can also choose to wake up. Wriggling the toes or holding the breath are both effective ways of waking up from a dream.

Calm, conscious breathing can help children to relax and watch their dream film. It is good to practice calming breathing techniques and associated affirmations with the child by day in a quiet, safe place, and suggest that she can do the same thing when she becomes lucid in a dream.[18] The child can also choose any short phrase which feels right: "I am safe"; "I am lucid"; "This is a beautiful dream." Sometimes, the usual visual elements of a dream are not present: when I was very young, I used to see a fiery luminescence filling up my bedroom as I went off to sleep. This is what I now consider to be the "Lucid Light;" the substance or energy from which dreams are created. Back then, I would simply watch in awe as this light surrounded me and lifted me into my dreams. When visuals are present, watching the dream film can help a child to understand the inner workings of her dream world and her personal dream signs—recurring motifs which crop up in her dreams. A familiarity with dream signs can trigger more lucid dreams as the child realizes: "A floating rabbit—I must be dreaming again!"

Go with the Flow

The second level of lucid dream magic happens during "Passive Participation Lucid Dreams."[19] Here, the dreamer goes with the flow of the dream action; joining in without trying to change or direct events. This is generally easier than remaining a passive, witnessing presence and watching the dream film, as dreams are multisensory, moving, three-dimensional immersive experiences that invite participation. Most children will automatically continue to engage with the dream when they become lucid, and this can feel exciting, like being an actor in your own fantasy film.

Here, the magic of knowledge that one is dreaming is mixed with super realistic sensory immersion and action. The lucid dreamer is fully part of the dream and experiences extraordinary things with all his senses and full conscious awareness: flying without wings; talking to grandma who died last year; healing from illness; meeting angels. Such lucid dreams can also give children insights into what may one day be possible, help them to experiment with different identities and ages, and rehearse new skills. In this dream reported by my daughter when she was four, she said that she knew she was dreaming. In telling the dream, she flung herself on the bed to show me how she had kicked her legs while swimming.

> *I dreamed about a big swimming pool and I was swimming with no swim noodle just like you, with nothing!*

Although it is perfectly possible for "go with the flow" lucid dreams to be calm experiences, my doctoral research found that this level of lucid dream engagement can result in daring dreams, involving actions such as skydiving or white-water rafting, which the dreamer has never experienced in waking life. Often lucidity is triggered when unusual sensations are experienced or when something astonishing or exhilarating happens. If the lucid dreamer hangs in there and goes with whatever is happening, free from fear, she may have one of the most wonderful dream experiences of her life. The difficulty for some dreamers is staying lucid throughout the maelstrom of sensory activity, so when tumbling over the edge of a waterfall or competing against dinosaurs in a sack race, it is useful to repeat from time to time: "This is a dream."

Touches of Magic

On the third level of lucid dream magic, the dreamer actively makes changes in the dream content, but only sporadically, which is why I term them Sporadic Control Lucid Dreams.[20] The dreamer delivers an initial impulse to the dream, such as asking a question of a dream figure or flying up into the sky. Then he relinquishes control and sees what happens next. This level allows the dreamer to guide the dream but it also allows the dream ample opportunity to respond with all the rich surprise of the unconscious. As if with a magic wand, the dreamer touches the dream and it transforms in surprising and insightful ways. This type of dream magic turns the lucid dream into a conscious conversation between the dreamer and the dream. For children, experimenting with lucid dream magic can be a thrilling game, and it can also be psychologically helpful to engage consciously with lucid dream figures, whether they seem nonthreatening or monstrous.

In Patricia Garfield's 1974 book *Creative Dreaming*, mention is made of the Senoi tribe's technique of asking frightening dream figures for a gift. Dreamworkers and lucid dream experts over decades have reported wonderful results with this technique.[21] Dreamworker and artist Sheila McNellis Asato reports her success with teaching it in classrooms:

> I ask if anyone has ever had a nightmare in which they have been chased, and of course many hands go up. I ask for a volunteer to tell their dream story to the group. We then act out the moment in which the dreamer is being chased and STOP, ask ourselves if we could be dreaming, then turn around and face whoever is chasing us and say in a loud voice, "Who are you? What do you want? What is your present for me?"
>
> The kids love to do this scenario over and over again. Practice through play is essential for reinforcing dream skills. Then the kids are told to go home, dream and report back the next day. Inevitably, someone will say that they tried the Senoi method and it worked![22]

There are many ways of applying touches of magic to a dream when lucid. These ideas for children's lucid dreams can be tweaked to make them age-appropriate. Rehearsing any which appeal to the child during the day, in a safe space, is helpful. In particular it is useful for the child to decide before bed whom to call on for help if he or she becomes lucid in a frightening dream.

- When you know you are dreaming, ask the dream to make a certain person or animal appear. Call your request out loud: "I'd like to see my hamster!" Then wait and see what the dream comes up with.
- Make something in the dream shrink small by pointing at it and saying: "Shrink!" Then see if the dream reacts. Something completely unexpected may happen. Every attempt at lucid dream experimentation teaches you more about the nature of your personal dream world.
- Summon help: if you are faced with something scary, call for your favorite cartoon character, stuffed toy or football/movie star to help you out. Super-heroes and parents work too! In a dream, help is always at hand. You just need to ask for it calmly and fully expect it to show up.
- Ask a dream figure what it wants. Ask if it has a gift for you. Give it a gift. If you have nothing to give, look around and say: "Under that stone I will find the perfect present for this dream figure." Then lift the stone.

Dream Wizardry

The fourth level of dream magic corresponds to what I have termed Continuous Control Lucid Dreams.[23] Even in the most determinedly con-trolled lucid dream, there always seem to be uncontrollable elements, so this level simply refers to lucid dreams where the dreamer *continuously attempts* to manipulate the dream throughout its duration. The dream itself will fill in details and generate surprise twists, so it seems safe to say that the natural spontaneity of the dream never disappears completely. Some people resist the idea of lucid dreaming as they fear it is all about controlling dreams and crushing potentially important unconscious messages. Yet if dreams have something important to tell us, they come back again and shout more and more loudly, as can be seen in the case of recurrent night-mares. Experienced lucid dreamers know that *not* influencing a lucid dream is all but impossible due to its thought-responsive nature.[24]

It can take many minutes and hours of lucid dreaming to learn this level of dream magic. On the other hand, children are such fast learners that when they become aware that something is possible, they can immediately get the hang of it. I familiarized my daughter with the concept of lucid dreaming and befriending dream monsters when she had dragon nightmares aged two and a quarter. The lucid dream at the start of this chapter falls into the "dream wizardry" category: When Yasmin was four, powerful dream witches began to bother her, wanting to gobble her up, and this dream marked the breakthrough moment when she used lucid magic to placate and befriend them.[25] Her amazement at the doll unexpectedly coming to life demonstrates the eternal creativity of the dream even when faced with the spells of a young wizard.

When might it be psychologically useful for children to attempt full dream control? Aside from the playful, experimental fun of it, and the intense happiness of starring in your own dream, dream wizardry could be helpful for children who feel powerless in their waking life, for those who have been suffering from nightmares, and for victims of trauma or abuse. Exercising their personal power in an environment from which they know they will awaken safely can help children to take the first step out of a victim mentality. British lucid dreamer Natalie O'Neill had recurring nightmares throughout her childhood. In the worst one, her sister was strapped to a conveyor belt in the sitting room and was moving toward an evil man who was waiting to get her. For years, this nightmare defeated the young Natalie because although she knew she was dreaming, she felt frozen to the spot and incapable of acting to save her sister. Then one night the penny dropped and she realized she *could* change the nightmare. She manifested a knife and stabbed the evil man. This first step from helpless bystander to somebody who could act to change terrible things empowered Natalie.[26] The nightmare never returned.

Here are some ideas to inspire and help apprentice dream wizards of all ages:

- Materialize a magic wand, a wishing ring, or an invisibility cloak, and see what they can do. Decide before you sleep which magical prop you would like to use, and strongly visualize it working.
- Make up a spell, either before you sleep or spontaneously when you next become lucid. Aged 4.5 my daughter reported this lucid dream and subsequently drew it with felt-tips and glitter as shown in Figure 14.1:

I was a fairy and I turned you and Daddy into fairies too and we had magic crowns and your crown was silver and we said: "Silver crown, silver crown! Fly us to the moon and stars and sun!" And it did.

- Paint a door by pointing your finger up, along and down in the shape of a door, then walk through it saying: "Through this door is a world full of ice cream!" Test out other commands and see how the dream responds.
- Transform yourself into a superhero and dash through the skies. If you see anyone or anything that needs help, use your powers to save them.

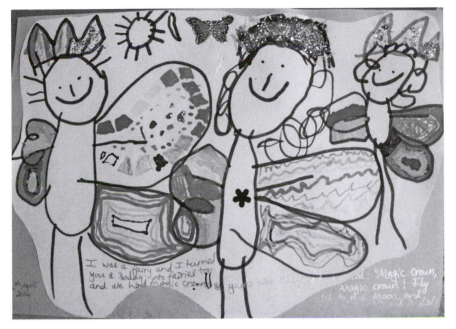

Figure 14.1   "Fly us to the Moon!" (Yasmin Johnson, age 4.5)

- Practice being the best in the world at something you love: beat on some drums, water-ski like a pro, pilot your own plane. Anything is possible! Bring the happy feeling back with you into your waking life.
- Turn yourself into an animal. Announce: "I am a tortoise!" or "Now I become a panda bear!"

Healing Nightmares: All You Need is L.O.V.E.

These aliens came to earth. They pretended to be friendly, then they attacked, killing everybody except me, then one ate me. It started on my hand and slowly worked upwards and I couldn't stop it. Each alien had pointed ears and small beady eyes in a head too big for its body.[27] (Donna, age 8)

Children have the most terrible nightmares in which they cannot stop events. They fall victim to witches, devils, out-of-control tractors and axe-wielding strangers. They have their skin pulled off or are attacked with chain saws.[28] They are annihilated again and again. If a child has nobody with whom to share a nightmare, or if a well-meaning parent dismisses bad dreams and makes it clear that what happens in dreams is not up for discussion, it is a safe bet that the nightmares will keep on coming. Although there is an understandable tendency on the part of sleep-deprived parents to view nightmares as purely negative events that need to be banned from the child's bedroom forever, nightmares harbor deep creative energy. Harnessing this energy can be both healing and empowering for children.

The idea that lucid dreaming could help children with nightmares is not new. Nearly a hundred years ago, back in 1921, Mary Arnold-Forster suggested that lucid dreaming techniques could be beneficial for children suffering from harrowing dreams.[29] In recent decades, studies have backed up such theories.[30] Psychotherapists increasingly report great successes with teaching children to resolve nightmares through lucid dreaming. One girl of 12 tried to save her little brother from being mauled by two dogs, and ended up being severely bitten herself. Afterwards, she had recurring nightmares about being chased by dogs and hiding fearfully behind a tree. Her therapist, J. Timothy Green, told her about lucid dreaming, and two weeks later she reported a lucid dream where she stepped out from behind the tree and ordered the aggressive dogs to turn into hot dogs. They did, and she ate them up. The nightmare never returned.[31]

My experience with my daughter Yasmin provided me with a road map through the rocky terrain of nightmares. I realized that the four most important things were to *Listen* when a child talks about dreams; provide the child with *Options*; *Verify* their progress; and *Empower* them. The L.O.V.E. nightmare empowerment technique was born, and it can be applied to any age group as long as age-appropriate suggestions are made.

The L.O.V.E. Nightmare Empowerment Technique

Listen

The "L" in L.O.V.E. is crucial. Listen to children when they share dreams and nightmares with you. Stop what you are doing and give them your full attention. This validates their experience and makes them aware that dreams are important. If you are unfamiliar with dreamwork, keep it simple—there is no need to feel obliged to try and interpret the dream or link it to waking life events. Expressing emotions and being heard is recognized to have powerful healing qualities even if no advice is offered.[32] Listening to the dream will have a therapeutic effect, so simply by listening you are helping the child because he knows he is being heard.

Options

Young dreamers need to be aware of their options. A child does not have to tolerate being eaten alive in a dream. A dream is not something that "just happens" to people: It is a cocreation generated by the interaction between the unconscious mind and the dreamer. Dreams are highly thought-responsive environments that react to the dreamer's thoughts, emotions, expectations, fears, and intentions. Options for children suffering from nightmares include all the possibilities available to a child when he or she becomes lucid within a dream. They also include all types of dreamplay, such as drawing or acting out the dream, which I view as a kind of "waking lucidity." All children need to know that they can ask for help in a dream and it will appear. They also need to know the "game over" option: They can wriggle their toes or hold their breath to wake up from a scary dream.

It can be enough to ask a child: "Would you like to draw the dream monster?" or to remark: "If a monster comes after you and you *know* that you are dreaming, you can ask him to be your friend instead of scaring you." With recurring nightmares, a higher level of engagement may be necessary. A young child and a trusted adult could try shouting together at the dream monster to GO AWAY!

Verify

Once the child has been listened to carefully and offered options for how to play with and transform the nightmare, it is important to verify his or her progress over the next few days or weeks. This does not mean that adults should hound the child for details; it is enough to be available and ask occasional questions if the moment seems right—when dream sharing at the breakfast table, a parent might ask, "Did that recurring nightmare ever come back?" Or simply: "Do you have a dream you'd like to talk about?" Therapists and educators will have clearly defined moments of time with children in which to discuss and further develop dreamplay. Verifying a child's progress with nightmares demonstrates your continuing interest in her welfare and allows you to help her to change tactics if need be.

Empower

Tell the child: "There will always be help in your dreams when you need it." Encourage children to find fresh options for engaging with nightmares if the one they have tried seems not to be working. Help them to find a personal dream mantra or a spell. It is important to let the dreamer choose the dream ally, spell, or dream equipment (a spaceship; a magic shell) that works best for him. Different nightmares may require different solutions. The child can practice these by day through acting them out or performing gestures such as "wrapping myself in protective white light that no monster can get through." After a talk about scary dreams, I suggested a mantra to my two-and-a-half-year-old. The next day I heard her shouting in her room. Looking in, I saw her jumping up and down on her bed, yelling at the top of her voice: "This is MY dream!" Talk about self-empowerment: She was all fired up with excitement at the thought of trying this out in her next bad dream. Soon there was no more mention of the sharp-toothed tiger that had been troubling her, and she reported dream solutions such as help arriving when she was scared.

Children react well to power objects: encourage them to slip a talismanic object under their pillow before bedtime, or make a dream catcher for their bedroom to keep bad dreams away. When a child believes, trusts, and eventually *knows from experience* that he can transform bad things into something good and befriend monsters, this can have a powerful effect on his psyche. The result can be increased confidence and the sense of being more at ease in the world.

Dreamplay as Waking Lucidity

Dreamplay refers to forms of dream-related waking activities that help dreamers to engage with their own dreams or the dreams of others. Sketching a dream is dreamplay. So is turning the energy of the dream into a dance, a piece of music, or a play. Dreamplay is like lucid dreaming because deep unconscious dream imagery and the alert, awake mind interact in symbiosis to cocreate something new and valuable. Elsewhere I have termed this highly beneficial interaction "Lucid Dreamplay."

Dreamplay with children should be child-led, which means it should never be forced: If a child does not want to draw her nightmare, do not push her. If a child doing dream theater is dead-set on slaughtering the dream monster, and you feel it would be more beneficial (and let's be honest, nicer) for her to befriend it, what should you do? I would advise letting her slaughter it if that is what she feels she needs to do. Killing the dream monster can do a great deal of psychological good as it propels the child out of a victim mentality. Once a child has proved to himself that he can destroy something terrifying, he may be more open to listening to other possibilities, such as asking it why it wanted to eat him, or if it has a message for him. He may want to take a turn at being the dream monster and speaking with its voice, and this empathy game can transform a child's perception of a dream monster completely and forever.

When dreamplay is guided with the basic precepts of kindness, acceptance, and empathy in mind, with love as the bottom line, it becomes another way of showing children ways of resolving waking life situations with the same moral compass. Try asking the child who has happily beaten a dream dragon to death in role play: "Now, is there any way of acting out that again, and seeing what happens if you open your arms to the dragon with love in your heart and ask him to be your friend?" Of course, it is fine if the child retorts, "No way!" Some nightmares are so horrible that initially it may take a while before a child feels safe and strong enough to do anything other than kill the enemy as fast as he or she can. It is good to offer options and allow the dreamplay to develop over time. Patience and kindness are key.

Soon enough, the effects of dreamplay will show up in a child's dreams. Giovani, a nine-year-old Bahamian boy, did dreamplay with Ann Wiseman on confronting nightmare monsters. He was experiencing recurring nightmares of being chased by a bear, and one night he reported waking suddenly after another encounter with the bear:

> *I felt desperate and thought I was going to die, so I woke up. Then I remembered what you said about drawing the dream and talking to the monster. Next time I went to sleep [the bear] came back and instead of running, I asked him why he was scaring me. He said he was just trying to get some attention. "Every time I go into someone's dream," he said, "they run away. . . . You are the first person who stood up to me. I have no one to talk to so I get very angry, now we are friends."[33]*

Imagine the solace of having a powerful dream bear as a friend! A living dream friend is worth more than a dead dream enemy. This same dream bear can now protect Giovani if he has scary dreams in the future. Children who manage to turn dream monsters into allies can be encouraged to honor this new friendship in any way that feels right for them, from drawing a picture of the two of them doing something fun together to making or buying a stuffed bear to put on their pillow at night.

Dreamplay Options for Adults to Share with Children

- Do not just draw the dream monster: draw help into your dream picture. This puts the focus on having the power to change feelings of powerlessness. Help might be a friendly wizard, a shield, a ladder, a strong parent, or a trapdoor that the monster falls through.
- Rehearse the following tricks to protect you in nightmares: Try a magic "be my friend" spell. Singing or chanting words can charge them with special power, as can rhymes. Pull a circle of white light around you so you feel safe and protected. Send love to a dream monster. Act out gestures of love and

friendship: hands over heart, or arms open wide. Shout a power word: anything from *abracadabra* to a Harry Potter spell, a poem, or a prayer.

- Create a "dream zoo" by drawing or modeling your dream monsters and dream animals. Make high-walled cages out of cardboard boxes. This is your zoo, so you get to make up the rules.
- Make a dream book. Use any materials you want to collage your dreams: felt-tips or watercolors, wool for fields, sequins for stars. Write the dream around your picture in circles, or jot down the main words that sum it up.
- Interview your dream figures. Find out how they feel and why they act the way they do.
- Create a magic dream box and put in any objects or drawings that represent helpful things or people from your dreams. A river stone could be the dream mountain. A chocolate wrapper could be the gold nugget you found in a dream. Look at these before you sleep to remind you of the treasures your dreams bring. Tonight will bring even more treasure!

The Lucid Writing Technique

I developed this technique in 2003 and it has since been tested in classrooms and workshops internationally and embraced by established therapists. A waking version of lucid dreaming, Lucid Writing[34] is a simple yet effective technique for exploring dreams. Children too young to write can try it verbally, while sitting or lying with eyes closed. Older children who can write fluently should practice the technique with a trusted adult at hand, as it can raise deep emotions, especially when a nightmare is worked with.

- Choose a recent dream, or one which is very vivid. Short dreams are best, or a dream with a strong central image or feeling.
- Close your eyes and bring your attention to your breath. With each exhale, relax a little more. Imagine yourself bathed in golden light, completely safe and relaxed.
- Now bring your dream image into your mind. Focus on it. Notice colors, shapes, feelings.
- The dream image might transform and turn into something else. You can guide this process in ways similar to the lucid dreaming techniques in this chapter—that is, you could have an internal "chat" with any dream figures, or ask for help. Or you can simply watch and see what happens.
- When you feel ready, open your eyes just slightly, enough to see your paper and pen. Then write without stopping and without worrying about what you are writing! Let the writing go wherever it wants to go.

In Lucid Writing, something surprising often happens to change the dream, like a turn in the river taking the dreamer not over the edge of a waterfall as he feared in his nightmare, but into a beautiful new world. The dream imagery mingles with waking consciousness to cocreate a new dream. Associations and insights into waking life situations may arise: "Oh—in this dream I feel just like I felt when my teacher yelled at me! Now I see that she was not so much angry as worried that I would hurt myself." It can be a transformative, healing experience, or simply an interesting dream game to play which teaches children how thoughts, feelings, dreams and the imagination can be mixed together to create streams of imagery. Lucid Writing can be great practice for lucid dreaming, as with minimal effort, vivid mental imagery can be guided and played with much as the lucid dreamer can play with the dream.

Dream Intelligence

Who is more likely to develop good self-esteem, creative thinking, and resourcefulness—the child being beaten down every night by nightmares she has no idea she can change, or the child who knows she can tame dragons in her lucid dreams, befriend scary witches, and swim like a dolphin?

When children are taught the potential of lucid dreaming, they are better equipped to summon the necessary courage and creativity we all need to get through the unpredictable situations of daily life. If children know the possibilities available to them when they become lucid in a dream, this knowledge empowers them. They can learn to act in their dreams and act in their lives toward greater personal happiness. When lucidity is mixed with waking dreamplay techniques, children gain a deeper understanding of their own inner source of wisdom, and as they learn to look within for answers, they are learning an important life skill.

Combining lucid dreaming with waking dreamplay can result in the development of empathy, mental flexibility, intuition, self-awareness, and resourcefulness. I call this mixture of skills "dream intelligence." Dream intelligence is not restricted to dreams; it carries over into waking life situations and becomes a tool for empowerment. Educators, parents, and caregivers can help nurture dream intelligence and trigger lasting positive changes in a child's dream life by guiding children through the possibilities open to them in the world of lucid dreaming and dreamplay. Transformation can be swift and powerful when this guidance is done with respect for the child's dreams, a playful approach, sound ethics, and a big dose of L.O.V.E.

So much of a child's dream life depends on the attitude the adults in their life have toward dreaming. As adults, we can open doors for children. The lucid dreaming door could enable a child to step into a creative, fulfilling dream life. As the dream life gets happier, so does waking life because the personality grows more balanced. If we can give one gift to the next generation, let it be the key to a happy, creative dream life!

But a key is useless if there is nobody there to turn it in the lock.

This is where you, the adult, step in. When you listen to children's dreams, when you take a child by the hand and guide him safely into dreamplay, when you show him the possibilities of lucid dreaming . . . the door swings open.

Notes

1. Clare R. Johnson, "The Role of Lucid Dreaming in the Process of Creative Writing," PhD thesis (University of Leeds, England, 2007).

2. Daniel Erlacher and Michael Schredl, "Practicing a Motor Task in a Lucid Dream Enhances Subsequent Performance: A Pilot Study," *The Sport Psychologist* 24, no. 2 (2010): 157–167.

3. Private correspondence with Claire Shticks and her mother, reproduced with permission, November 28, 2014.

4. Antonio Zadra and R. O. Pihl, "Lucid Dreaming as a Treatment for Recurrent Nightmares," *Psychotherapy and Psychosomatics* 66, no. 1 (1997): 50–55; Victor Spoormaker, Jan van den Bout, and Eli J. G. Meijer, "Lucid Dreaming Treatment for Nightmares: A Series of Cases," *Dreaming* 13, no. 3 (2003): 181–186.

5. Charles Tart, *States of Consciousness* (Authors Guild Backinprint.com Edition. Lincoln, NE: iUniverse.com, 2000), 54.

6. N. Lapina, V. Lysenko, and A. Burikov, "Age-Dependent Dreaming: Characteristics of Secondary School Pupils," *Sleep Supplement* 21 (1998): 287.

7. X. Qinmei, L. Qinggong, and L. Jie, "4–6 Year Old Children's Understanding of the Origins and Controllability of Dreams," *Acta Psychologica Sinica* 38, no. 1 (2006): 70–78.

8. Paul Tholey and Kaleb Utecht, *Schöpferisch Träumen: Der Klartraum als Lebenshilfe* (Frankfurt: Klotz [1995] 2008).

9. Patricia Garfield, *Creative Dreaming* (New York: Ballantine Books, [1976] 1988).

10. Stephen LaBerge, *Lucid Dreaming* (New York: Ballantine Books, 1985).

11. Clare R. Johnson, "Magic, Meditation, and the Void: Creative Dimensions of Lucid Dreaming," in *Lucid Dreaming: New Perspectives on Consciousness in Sleep*, eds. Ryan Hurd and Kelly Bulkeley (Santa Barbara, CA: Praeger, 2014).

12. Brenda Mallon, *Dream Time with Children* (London: Jessica Kingsley Publishers, 2002).

13. Johnson, "Role of Lucid Dreaming."

14. Clare R. Johnson, "Lucid Dreaming in the Creative Process," paper presented at the *22nd Conference of the International Association for the Study of Dreams*, June 24–28, Berkeley, CA, 2005.

15. Johnson, "Magic, Meditation, Void."

16. Clare R. Johnson, "Lucid Dream Your Way to Creativity," paper presented at the *IASD Fourth Psiber Dreaming Conference*, September 18–October 2 2005; Johnson, "Role of Lucid Dreaming," 18.

17. Celia Green and Charles McCreery, *Lucid Dreaming: The Paradox of Consciousness during Sleep* (London: Routledge, 1994), 132.

18. http://deepluciddreaming.com/childrens-lucid-dreams-and-nightmares.

19. Johnson, "Role of Lucid Dreaming," 22.

20. Ibid., 24.

21. Ann Sayre Wiseman, *The Nightmare Solution* (San Francisco, USA: Echo Point Books, 2013); Garfield: *Creative Dreaming*; LaBerge, *Lucid Dreaming*.

22. Private interview with Sheila McNellis Asato; www.monkeybridgearts.com.

23. Johnson, "Role of Lucid Dreaming," 27.

24. Clare R. Johnson, "Surfing the Rainbow: Fearless and Creative out-of-Body Experiences," in Alexander De Foe (ed.) *Consciousness beyond the Body: Evidence and Reflections* (Melbourne: Centre for Exceptional Human Potential, 2016); Johnson, "Magic, Meditation, Void."

25. Clare R. Johnson, "Children's Lucid Dreams & Nightmares: Taming Dragons and Witches through Lucid Dreaming," YouTube video: http://deeplucid dreaming.com/2015/10/childrens-nightmares-how-lucid-dreaming-can-help/.

26. Private interview with Natalie O'Neill, 2014.

27. Donna, 8, in Mallon, *Dream Time with Children*, 87.

28. Mallon, *Dream Time with Children*; Wiseman, *The Nightmare Solution*.

29. Mary Arnold-Forster, *Studies in Dreams* (London: Allen and Unwin, 1921).

30. H. Abramovitch, "The Nightmare of Returning Home: A Case of Acute Onset Nightmare Disorder Treated by Lucid Dreaming," *Israel Journal of Psychiatry Related Sciences* 32, no. 2 (1995): 140–145; A. Brylowski, "Nightmare in Crisis: Clinical Applications of Lucid Dreaming Techniques," *Psychiatric Journal of the University of Ottawa* 15, no. 2 (1990): 79–84; Zadra and Pihl, "Lucid Dreaming Recurrent Nightmares"; Spoormaker et al., "Lucid Dreaming Treatment."

31. J. Timothy Green, "Lucid Dreaming in the Treatment of Post-Traumatic Stress Disorder," http://www.world-of-lucid-dreaming.com/lucid-dreaming-in -the-treatment-of-post-traumatic-stress-disorder.html.

32. James W. Pennebaker, *Opening Up: The Healing Power of Expressing Emotions* (New York, Guilford Press, 1997).

33. Wiseman, *Nightmare Solution*, 14.

34. Johnson, "Role of Lucid Dreaming," 36.

Bibliography

Abramovitch, H. "The Nightmare of Returning Home: A Case of Acute Onset Nightmare Disorder Treated by Lucid Dreaming." *Israel Journal of Psychiatry Related Sciences* 32, no. 2 (1995): 140–145.

Arnold-Forster, Mary. *Studies in Dreams*. London: Allen and Unwin, 1921.

Brylowski, A. "Nightmare in Crisis: Clinical Applications of Lucid Dreaming Techniques." *Psychiatric Journal of the University of Ottawa* 15, no. 2 (1990): 79–84.

Erlacher, Daniel, and Michael Schredl. "Practicing a Motor Task in a Lucid Dream Enhances Subsequent Performance: A Pilot Study." *The Sport Psychologist* 24, no. 2 (2010): 157–167.

Garfield, Patricia. *Creative Dreaming*. New York: Ballantine Books, [1976] 1988.

Green, Celia, and Charles McCreery. *Lucid Dreaming: The Paradox of Consciousness during Sleep*. London, Routledge, 1994.

Johnson, Clare R. "Lucid Dreaming in the Creative Process." Paper presented at the *22nd Conference of the International Association for the Study of Dreams*, June 24–28, Berkeley, CA, 2005.

Johnson, Clare R. "Lucid Dream Your Way to Creativity." Paper presented at the *IASD Fourth Psiber Dreaming Conference*, September 18–October 2, 2005.

Johnson, Clare R. "The Role of Lucid Dreaming in the Process of Creative Writing." PhD thesis, University of Leeds, England, 2007.

Johnson, Clare R. "Magic, Meditation, and the Void: Creative Dimensions of Lucid Dreaming." In *Lucid Dreaming: New Perspectives on Consciousness in Sleep*, eds. Ryan Hurd and Kelly Bulkeley. Santa Barbara, CA: Praeger, 2014.

Johnson, Clare R. "Children's Lucid Dreams & Nightmares: Taming Dragons and Witches through Lucid Dreaming." YouTube video: http://deepluciddreaming .com/2015/10/childrens-nightmares-how-lucid-dreaming-can-help/.

Johnson, Clare R. "Surfing the Rainbow: Fearless and Creative out-of-Body Experiences." In De Foe, A. (ed.), *Consciousness beyond the Body: Evidence and Reflections*. Melbourne: Centre for Exceptional Human Potential, 2016.

LaBerge, Stephen. *Lucid Dreaming*. New York: Ballantine Books, 1985.

Lapina, N., V. Lysenko, and A. Burikov. "Age-Dependent Dreaming: Characteristics of Secondary School Pupils." *Sleep Supplement* 21, 1998.

Mallon, Brenda. *Dream Time with Children*. London: Jessica Kingsley Publishers, 2002.

Pennebaker, James W. *Opening Up: The Healing Power of Expressing Emotions*. New York: Guilford Press, 1997.

Qinmei, X., L. Qinggong, and L. Jie. "4–6 Year Old Children's Understanding of the Origins and Controllability of Dreams." *Acta Psychologica Sinica* 38, no. 1 (2006): 70–78.

Spoormaker, Victor, Jan van den Bout, and Eli Meijer. "Lucid Dreaming Treatment for Nightmares: A Series of Cases." *Dreaming* 13, no. 3 (2003): 181–186.

Tart, Charles. *States of Consciousness*. Lincoln, NE: Authors Guild Backinprint.com Edition, iUniverse.com, 2000.

Tholey, Paul and Kaleb Utecht. *Schöpferisch Träumen: Der Klartraum als Lebenshilfe*. Frankfurt: Klotz, [1995] 2008.

Wiseman, Ann Sayre. *The Nightmare Solution*. San Francisco, USA: Echo Point Books, 2013.

Zadra, Antonio, and R. O. Pihl. "Lucid Dreaming as a Treatment for Recurrent Nightmares." *Psychotherapy and Psychosomatics* 66, no. 1 (1997): 50–55.

Resources

Books for Adult Readers about Dreams and Sleep

Dreams

Adams, Kate. *Unseen Worlds: Looking Through the Lens of Childhood*. London: Jessica Kingsley Publishers, 2010.
Unseen Worlds explores not only dreams but the vast imaginal worlds of children; their fears, coping strategies, and how they learn through play.

Barrett, Deirdre. *The Committee of Sleep: How Artists, Scientists and Athletes Use Their Dreams for Creative Problem Solving, and How You Can Too*. New York: Crown, 2001.
This book draws together examples throughout the ages of people utilizing their dreams for creativity. An encouraging, fascinating book for those who want to learn how to act on their dreams.

Beaudet, Denyse. *Dreamguider: Open the Door to Your Child's Dreams*. Charlottesville, VA: Hampton Roads Publishing Company, 2008.
Jungian developmental psychologist helps parents understand their dreams by engaging in their dream world.

Bulkeley, Kelly and Alan J. Siegel. *Dreamcatching: Every Parent's Guide to Exploring and Understanding Children's Dreams and Nightmares*. New York: Three Rivers Press, 1998.
Wonderful and useful guide for parents working with a child's dreams and nightmares.

Bynum, Edward Bruce. *Families and the Interpretation of Dreams*. New York: Haworth Press, 1993.
Shows how dreams reflect family life, giving case examples.

Cartwright, Rosalind and Lamberg, Lynne. *Crisis Dreaming: Using Your Dreams to Solve Your Problems*. London: Aquarian, 1993.

A valuable guide to how dreams can help those coping with life crises such as divorce, bereavement, illness, or job loss.

Epel, Naomi. *Writers Dreaming*. New York: Vintage, 1994.
In this insightful book, 26 writers talk about how their dreams connect with their creative process.

Garfield, Patricia. *Creative Dreaming*. New York: Ballantine, 1976.
This classic introduction to dreams examines a wide range of dream examples and gives tips for dealing with nightmares.

Garfield, Patricia. *Your Child's Dreams*. New York: Ballantine, 1984.
This is a book full of many resources for parents and others who want to understand a child's dream life.

Jay, Clare [Clare R. Johnson]. *Breathing in Colour*. London: Piatkus, 2009.
A lucid-dream-inspired novel about a mother's search through India for her teenaged daughter who went missing while backpacking.

Johnson, Clare R. *Llewellyn's Complete Book of Lucid Dreaming: A Comprehensive Guide to Promote Creativity, Overcome Sleep Disturbances & Enhance Health and Wellness*. Minnesota: Llewellyn Worldwide, 2017.
An in-depth, practical guide to all aspects of lucid dreaming ranging from problem-solving and creativity to children's lucid dreams and nightmare solutions.

L'Engle, Medeline. *Walking on Water*. New York: Farrar, 1972.
An investigation of the world of dreams and imagination by an award-winning children's author.

Mallon, Brenda. *Dreamtime with Children*. London: Jessica Kingsley Publishers, 2002.
This excellent book has resources and information for understanding children's dreams and ideas for working with children to assist them to remember and enjoy their dreams.

Mellick, Jill. *The Natural Artistry of Dreams*. Berkeley: Conari Press, 1996.
A dreamplay resource book par excellence, Mellick's book explores everything from making dream masks and mandalas to active imagination. Most of her techniques and ideas can be done with children of all ages.

Sunderland, Margot. *Using Story Telling as a Therapeutic Tool with Children*. London: Speechmark, 2000.
For parents and caregivers who would like practical guidance on how to help traumatized, frightened, and overwhelmed children to develop inner resources through storytelling.

Waggoner, Robert. *Lucid Dreaming: Gateway to the Inner Self*. Needham, MA: Moment Point Press, 2009.
A personal journey into lucid dreaming and a great general guide to the subject.

Wiseman, Ann Sayre. *Nightmare Help for Children.* San Francisco: Ten Speed Press, 1986.

A hard-to-find book that teaches adults ways to help children discover their own understanding of a dream.

Sleep and Sleep Disorders

Conesa Sevilla, Jorge. *Wrestling with Ghosts: A Personal and Scientific Account of Sleep Paralysis.* Bloomington, IN: Xlibris Corporation, 2004.

A personal account of sleep paralysis and how to enter lucid dreams from this state.

Dement, William and Christopher Vaughn. *The Promise of Sleep.* New York: Random House, 2009.

Best-selling book about sleep health by Stanford professor W. Dement, who is considered "the father of sleep medicine."

Ekirch, A. Roger. *At Day's Close: Night in Times Past.* New York: Norton, 2005.

Wonderfully written history of the night, including perspectives on sleep and dreams since the early modern period.

Hurd, Ryan. *Sleep Paralysis: A Guide to Hypnagogic Visions and Visitors of the Night.* San Mateo: Enlightened Hyena Press, 2011.

Guidebook for managing and learning to thrive with sleep paralysis and its attendant dreamlike visions.

Jay, Clare [Clare R. Johnson]. *Dreamrunner.* London: Piatkus, 2010.

The author's second lucid-dream-inspired novel explores the dark side of sleep, with the plot built around a mysterious sleep disorder that drives a gentle man to terrorize his family by night.

Naiman, Rubin. *Healing Night: The Science and Spirit of Sleeping, Dreaming and Awakening.* Minneapolis: Syren Book Company, 2006.

A healing book that considers sleep medicine from a holistic perspective, respecting the biological as well as the psycho-spiritual.

Schenck, Carlos. M.D. *SLEEP: A Groundbreaking Guide to the Mysteries, the Problems and the Solutions.* New York: Avery, 2007.

A fascinating resource for adults interested in the outer margins of sleep, including sleep disorders ranging from sleepwalking and night terrors to sleep-eating.

Books about Dreams for Readers Under 12

Abell, Angel Morgan. *The Alphabliss of Miss.* Chico, CA: Morgan Foundation Publishers, 2005.

This book offers children 26 alphabetical poems and pictures about magical dream allies that are girls with strong, unique, and empowering qualities.

Brown, Margaret Wise. *Goodnight Moon*. New York: Harper and Row, 1947.
    The perfect bedtime story for young children, as we say goodnight to the world.

Brown, Margaret Wise. *My World*. New York: Harper Festival, 2003.
    A beautiful companion book to the classic *Goodnight Moon*, seeing the big world through the eyes of a little bunny, for ages 1–4.

De Saint-Exupéry, Antoine. *The Little Prince*. New York: Harcourt, Brace and World, 1943.
    The classic story of the little space aviator who lands on earth is touching for all ages but parents of younger children should be aware of the sad ending.

Fox, Karen C. *Older than the Stars*. Watertown, MA: Charlesbridge, 2011.
    The story of the origins of the universe told with beautiful illustrations and simple yet informative prose is perfect for ages 7–10.

Frances, Renee. *A Visit from the Goodnight Fairy*. Victoria, BC: Friesen Press, 2014.
    This storybook is designed to help children under five to look forward to their dreams and fall asleep with ease.

Garrison, Christian. *The Dream Eater*. New York: MacMillan, 1978.
    This Japanese tale is meant to help children overcome their fear of scary dream figures.

Haddix, Margaret Peterson. *Found*. New York: Simon & Schuster Books for Young Readers, 2009.
    First book in *The Missing* series, *Found* is for the 8- to 12-year-olds who like time traveling and a bit of mystery and adventure thrown in with their sci-fi.

Harris, Annaka. *I Wonder*. Cleveland, OH: Four Elephants Press, 2013.
    Beautifully illustrated, *I Wonder* captures the conversation between a little girl and her mother who explore the great mysteries of life; appropriate for ages one and up.

Joyce, William. *The Man in the Moon*. New York: Simon & Schuster, Atheneum Books for Young Readers, 2011.
    A story for children about the man in the moon, who was once a child. He learned how to help other children with their fear of the dark by shining brightly in the night.

Law, Stephen. Illustrator Nishant Choksi. *Really, Really Big Questions: About Life, the Universe and Everything*. London: Kingfisher, 2012.
    A cool interactive book filled with brainteasers, quizzes, and bold illustrations to capture the imagination of any budding scientists age 7–12.

McNulty, Faith. *If You Decide To Go to the Moon*. New York: Scholastic Press, 2005.
    What would it be like to journey to the moon? This book is filled with space traveling fun facts for budding scientists and sci-fi fans ages 4–7 years.

Rees, Gwyneth. *Fairy Dreams: A Magical Journey to Fairyland*. London: Macmillan Children's Books, 2005.

A sensitive, magical book about a little girl whose grandmother dies, and how dreams (and fairies!) help her to connect with her and accept her death. Perfect to read aloud to six-year-olds.

Sendak, Maurice. *In the Night Kitchen*. New York: Harper and Row, 1970.

A young boy's dream journey through a surreal baker's kitchen.

Sendak, Maurice. *Where the Wild Things Are*. London: Random House, 2007.

After being sent to bed without his supper, Max dreams of the Island of the Wild Things.

Storr, Catherine. *Marianne Dreams*. London: Faber and Faber, 2006.

Bedridden with a long-term illness, Marianne dreams inside a picture she has drawn.

Wahl, Jan. *Humphrey's Bear*. New York: Henry Holt and Co., 1987, 2005.

A story for little ones who sleep with a furry toy animal that helps them not be afraid of the scary things at night.

White, E. B. *Stuart Little*. New York: Harper & Brothers, 1945.

This award-winning children's story was based on a dream.

Dream-Inspired Books for Young Adults

Card, Orson Scott. *Ender's Game*. New York, TOR, 1977.

Ender Wiggin changes the dream that changes the game.

Hubert, Cam. *Dreamspeaker*. New York, Avon, 1978.

The deeply moving story of a boy caught between two worlds. Set in British Columbia.

L'Engle, Madeleine. *A Wrinkle in Time*. Square Fish, 50 Anniversary Edition, 2012.

The first book in the *Time* trilogy, this time-bending classic and Newberry award winner is a perfect sci-fi introduction for preteens.

Patterson, Katherine. *Bridge to Terabithia*. New York: Avon, 1977.

Jess's friendship with Leslie and the worlds of imagination she opens to him, change forever.

Paulson, Gary. *The Night the White Deer Died*. New York: Laurel Leaf Library, 1978.

Janet, one of the few Anglo teens in her community, begins having nightmares.

Pullman, Philip. *His Dark Materials Trilogy*. New York: Laurel Leaf, 2003.

This award winning trilogy focuses on two children who travel through parallel universes. Though recommended for young readers ages 12 and up, adults will appreciate the sophisticated underpinnings of physics, philosophy, and theology.

Storm, Hyemeyohsts. *Seven Arrows*. New York: Ballantine, 1972.
　　An adventure of the Plains Indian people and the Medicine Way.

Walker, Alice. *The Colour Purple*. New York: Harcourt Brace Jovanovich, 1982.
　　Walker repeatedly dreamed the "ancestors" who are characters in the book.

Wooten, Victor L. *The Music Lesson*. New York: Berkley Books, 2006.
　　From the Grammy-award winning bassist, a musical tale.

Wynne Jones, Diana. *Howl's Moving Castle*. New York: Harper-Collins Children's Books, 1986.
　　A warmhearted blend of humor, magic, and romance.

For Those Facing Illness, Trauma, or Bereavement

Books for Adults

Anderson, Frances E. *Art-Centered Education and Therapy for Children With Disabilities*. Springfield, IL: Charles C. Thomas, 1996.

Davenport, Leslie. *Healing and Transformation Through Guided Imagery*. Berkeley: Celestial Arts, 2009.

Garfield, Patricia L. *The Healing Power of Dreams*. New York: Simon and Schuster, 1991.

Klein, Nancy. *Healing Images for Children: Facing Cancer and Other Serious Illness*. Watertown WI: Inner Coaching, 2001.

Lasley, Justina. *Wake Up to Your Dreams*. Charleston, SC: Double Spiral Publishing, 2015.

Lyons, Tallulah. *Dreams and Guided Imagery: Gifts for Transforming Illness and Crisis*. Bloomington, IN: Balboa Press, 2012.

Mallon, Brenda. *Dreams, Counselling and Healing*. London: Gill and MacMillan, 2000.
　　Shows how dreams have been used in revealing illness and disease as well as offering potential healing pathways.

Mallon, Brenda. *Working with Bereaved Children and Young People*. Los Angeles: Sage, 2011.
　　Deals specifically with the impact of bereavement on children's dreams and shows how adults can help with the mourning process.

Naparstek, Belleruth. *Staying Well With Guided Imagery*. New York: Time Warner Books, 1994.

Norment, Rachel. *Guided by Dreams: Breast Cancer, Dreams and Transformation*. Richmond: Brandylane Publishers, 2006.

Resnick, Charlotte. *The Power of Your Child's Imagination: How to Transform Stress and Anxiety into Joy and Success.* New York: Penguin Group, 2009.

Rossman, Martin L., M.D. *Guided Imagery for Self-Healing.* New York: New World Library, 2000.

Zeltzer, Lonnie K. and Christina B. Schlank. *Conquering Your Child's Chronic Pain: A Pediatrician's Guide for Reclaiming a Normal Childhood.* New York: Harper Collins, 2005.
Recommended to parents with hospitalized children.

Books for Children

Bryan, Jenny. *What's Wrong with Me? What Happens When You're Sick and How to Stay Healthy.* New York: Thomas Learning, 1995.
Great illustrations. For grade school children.

Garvy, Helen. *Coping with Illness.* Los Gatos, CA: Shire Press, 1995.

For Teenagers with Serious Illness

Heegaard, Marge. *When Someone Has a Very Serious Loss or Illness: Children Can Cope with Loss and Change.* Minneapolis: Woodland Press, 1991.
Workbook used with children at cancer centers.

Mills, Joyce. Illustrator Brian Sebern, *Little Tree: A Story for Children with Serious Medical Problems.* Washington, DC: Magination Press, 2002.
For grade school children.

Shapiro, Lawrence E. and Robin K. Sprague. *The Relaxation and Stress Reduction Workbook for Kids.* Oakland, CA: Instant Help Books, 2009.

Websites and Online Resources for Dreams, Sleep, and Healing

American Sleep Apnea Association. Website: http://sleepapnea.org/treat/test-yourself.html
Self-tests if you think you are suffering from obstructive sleep apnea or some other sleep breathing disorder.

Child Life Specialists. Website: http://www.childlife.org

Deep Lucid Dreaming: Website: http://www.deepluciddreaming.com
Dr. Clare Johnson's website and blog explores all aspects of lucid dreaming, including children's lucid dreams and nightmares. Clare can be contacted here for advice.

The Healing Mind. Website: http://www.thehealingmind.org

Dr. Martin Rossman offers constructive advice about the power of the mind to heal illness.

The Healing Power of Dreams. Website: http://www.healingpowerofdreams.com
The website of Tallulah Lyons and Wendy Pannier, this site includes MP3 downloads of guided imagery for children and adults.

Health Journeys: Website: http://www.healthjourneys.com
Belleruth Naparstek's website provides a wealth of information about health and wellness modalities.

Imagery for Kids. Website: http://www.imageryforkids.com
Charlotte Resnick's website contains a load of helpful suggestions for kids.

International Association for the Study of Dreams. Website: http://www.asdreams.org
The world's leading organization for dream study contains a wealth of information on dreams.

Juvenile Diabetes. Website: http://www.t1everydaymagic.com/diabetes-art-projects-to-do-with-your-child/

Lucid Living: www.wedreamnow.info
Dr. Beverly D'Urso's website explores living life as a lucid dream with its practical and spiritual implications.

Night Terror Resource Center. Website: http://www.nightterrors.org
The purpose of this site is to help people understand that there are medical solutions and reasons for night terrors.

World of Lucid Dreaming. Website: http://world-of-lucid-dreaming.com
This website has hundreds of helpful articles about promoting and working with lucid dreams.

"Children's Lucid Dreams: Taming Witches and Dragons through Lucid Dreaming," by Dr. Clare Johnson, filmed at the Dream Research Institute, London, 2014. http://deepluciddreaming.com/2015/10/childrens-nightmares-how-lucid-dreaming-can-help/
A short video where the speaker shares tips on how to empower children to resolve nightmares through lucid dreaming.

Index

About the Editors and Contributors

Editors

Clare R. Johnson, PhD, Board Director for the International Association for the Study of Dreams, and the first person to do a PhD on lucid dreaming as a creative writing tool (University of Leeds, UK), for over a decade Clare has spoken at conferences and international multimedia platforms on the role of lucid dreaming in creativity, healing, and dying. Author of *Llewellyn's Complete Book of Lucid Dreaming: A Comprehensive Guide to Promote Creativity, Overcome Sleep Disturbances & Enhance Health and Wellness*, she has also written two lucid-dream-inspired novels, *Breathing in Colour* and *Dreamrunner*, under her novelist name of Clare Jay.

Clare's L.O.V.E. nightmare empowerment technique helps children to work out nightmare solutions, while Lucid Writing can help older children and adults to dissolve creative blocks, transform nightmares, and initiate healing. Articles and videos on dreams and lucidity can be found on her website where she also responds to those seeking advice. www.DeepLucid Dreaming.com.

Jean M. Campbell, MA, is editor of the International Association for the Study of Dreams' (IASD) *Dream Time Magazine*, and a member of that organization's board of directors. She has also served as the Chair of IASD's Board and as President. An internationally known author, she developed a therapeutic model for working with dreams, DreamWork/BodyWork, which she teaches through the 501(c)3 nonprofit organization she directs, the iMAGE Project.

Jean founded the World Dreams Peace Bridge in 2001. This international group of dreamers has raised funds for war-traumatized children and created, along with children in Baghdad, Iraq, the "Crystal Birds Dream

Program" discussed in this book. She has taught literature and creative writing, and worked as a senior science fiction editor and publicist.

Contributors

Kate Adams, PhD (UK), Kate is head of research at Bishop Grosseteste University, Lincoln, UK. Her research specialism is children's spirituality and its relationship to education, with a specific interest in children's spiritual dreams. She is author of *Unseen Worlds: Looking Through the Lens of Childhood* (2010). In the book, she encourages readers to recognize the importance of worlds that children inhabit, both positive and negative, including their encounters in dreams and nightmares.

Arielle Boyes, BA (Canada), Arielle recently completed an Honors Psychology undergraduate degree at Grant MacEwan University. She plans to pursue a PhD in clinical psychology.

Kelly Bulkeley, PhD (USA), Visiting Scholar at the Graduate Theological Union, former President of the International Association for the Study of Dreams, and Senior Editor of *Dreaming*. His books include *Dreaming Beyond Death* (2006) and *Children's Dreams* (2011) (both with his mother Patricia M. Bulkley), *Dreaming in the Classroom* (with Philip King and Bernard Welt, 2011), *Lucid Dreaming* (with Ryan Hurd, 2014), and *Big Dreams* (2016). He is director of the Sleep and Dream Database (SDDb), a digital archive and search engine.

Patricia M. Bulkley, DMin (USA), is a former Chaplain and spiritual services provider for Hospice of Marin. She earned her doctor of ministry from Princeton Theological Seminary, and taught classes in pastoral care and counseling for many years at San Francisco Theological Seminary. She is coauthor with her son Kelly Bulkeley of *Dreaming Beyond Death* (2006) and *Children's Dreams* (2012).

Carson Flockhart, BA (Canada), Carson is a recent graduate of MacEwan University in Edmonton, Alberta. There he had the privilege of working and studying under Dr. Jayne Gackenbach and conducting research on video games and dreams, specifically in the area of nightmares. This research was recently presented at the Towards a Science of Consciousness Conference in 2015. Carson has been an avid player of video games since his youth and has acquired experience in all types of genres and platforms.

Jayne Gackenbach, PhD (Canada), is one of the past presidents of the International Association for the Study of Dreams, and a long-time dream researcher. For the first half of her career she did research into lucid dreaming and now does research into the effects of the use of digital media on dreams. She is the editor of *Conscious Mind, Sleeping Brain* and *Video Game Play and Consciousness*.

Patricia Garfield, PhD (USA), is a renowned dream expert and prize-winning author of 11 books on dreams. Her best seller *Creative Dreaming* (1974, 1995) is considered a classic and appears in 15 languages. She is a cofounder and past-president of the International Association for the Study of Dreams and received that organization's 2012 Lifetime Achievement Award. http://www.creativedreaming.org.

David Gordon, PhD (USA), is a Clinical Psychologist offering treatment for adolescents and adults at Studio for the Healing Arts in Norfolk, Virginia. Through his Dreamwork Institute, David conducts dream sharing groups, workshops, and retreats nationally and internationally throughout the United States and Canada. He has written extensively on dreams including his book *Mindful Dreaming* that explores elements of the Mythic Journey as well as lessons in mindfulness as they are reflected in our dreams.

Ryan Hurd, MA (USA), is a researcher, educator, and author. Ryan has written several books on dreaming and is most recently coeditor of *Lucid Dreaming: New Perspectives on Consciousness in Sleep* (2014). His peer-reviewed papers investigate nootropics for lucid dreaming, as well as the application of lucid dreaming and environmental hermeneutics for uncovering researcher novelty. Ryan is the founder of DreamStudies.org, dedicated to the public education about sleep, dreams, and imagination studies.

Tallulah Lyons, MEd (USA), is a former special education consultant and currently facilitates dream groups and workshops in two cancer centers in Atlanta, Georgia. She is a cofounder of an IASD project to bring dreamwork into integrative medicine facilities and has worked to bring dream groups into church settings. She is the author of *Dream Prayers: Dreams as a Spiritual Path* and *Dreams and Guided Imagery: Gifts for Transforming Illness and Trauma*.

Brenda Mallon, MEd, Adv. Diploma Counselling (UK), Brenda is an author, counselor, and TV presenter. Throughout her career she has specialized in dreams, believing them to hold the key to health and creativity.

Her 17 books include *Dreams, Counselling and Healing, The Dream Bible,* and *Working with Bereaved Children and Young People.* She made "Children Dreaming," a groundbreaking film for the BBC and was elected to the board of the International Association for the Study of Dreams in 2000.

Linda Mastrangelo, MA, LMFT (USA), is an author, educator, artist, and psychotherapist with a private practice in the San Francisco Bay area specializing in dreams and grief. She writes extensively on dreams for numerous publications, presents her award-winning work internationally and facilitates trainings and workshops for mental health professionals. Linda serves on the board of directors for the International Association for the Study of Dreams, is editor of *Dream News* and lives with her husband in the mystical Santa Cruz Mountains.

Angel Morgan, PhD (USA), completed the Dream Studies and Creativity Studies programs at Saybrook University. She holds an MA in human development and a BA in theater, film, and television. Dr. Morgan is founder of the Dreambridge.com, and on the advisory board for DreamsCloud.com. She teaches interdisciplinary Dreambridge seminars and co-instructs a course on Extraordinary Dreams with Stanley Krippner, PhD. Her research can be found on academia.edu, and her blog about dreams on the *Huffington Post.*

Ann Sinyard (Canada), was born and raised in Fort McMurray, Alberta, Canada. She graduated from MacEwan University and majored in psychology. At MacEwan she completed research with a new piece of technology, the Oculus Rift virtual reality goggles. This research was on the relationship between dreams and virtual reality video game play. Her future career goals include integrating virtual reality therapy with couples and family counseling.

Caterina Snyder (Canada), is an entrepreneur, author, artist, and blogger who currently resides in Edmonton, Alberta, Canada. She did her graduate work in business at Syracuse University and undergraduate work at the University of Alberta. She has lived and worked in both Canada and the United States and recently launched a freelance consulting business. Learn more at www.caterinasnyder.com or connect with her via Facebook, Instagram, Pinterest, or LinkedIn.

Martha A. Taylor, MSN (USA), was born in northwest Indiana, and raised in a family of ten. She practiced nursing, mainly with children, in hospitals in the United States, East Africa, and did relief work in Lebanon. She started two Home Health Agencies and worked in home health for several years. She has a deep interest in exploring consciousness through dance, body-work, dreams, and play! She lives with her partner in a small community in Virginia.

Dani Vedros, LCSW (USA), is a psychotherapist and workshop leader in Norfolk, Virginia. She has been in private practice for over 10 years. She has presented locally and nationally and has led many groups and workshops on the topics of dreams, spirituality, and healing. Prior to starting private practice, Dani worked for over 10 years providing psychotherapy to children and adolescents with severe mental health issues both in residential and community-based settings.